LDL...The Silent Killer

A No-nonsense Approach to Preventing Heart Disease and Stroke

Max L. Fields, M.D.

ISBN 0-7414-3136-X

Published by:

INFI∞ITY
PUBLISHING.COM

1094 New DeHaven Street, Suite 100
West Conshohocken, PA 19428-2713
Info@buybooksontheweb.com
www.buybooksontheweb.com
Toll-free (877) BUY BOOK
Local Phone (610) 941-9999
Fax (610) 941-9959

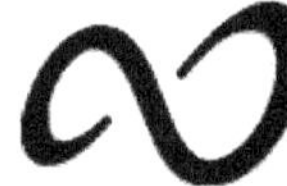

Printed in the United States of America

Printed on Recycled Paper

Published June 2006

Dedication

This book is dedicated to my friend, buddy, lover and wife, Betty.

Thanks loads to Deb Lindley and my wife, Betty. The office would surely have collapsed around me without you two.

Thanks to my great office staff who served so faithfully over the years. You are all so appreciated.

Thanks also to the staff of White County Memorial Hospital. We shared a lot of laughs and a lot of tears.

Thanks to my great consultants. Learning has been a continual joy.

Last but not least, thanks to my great patients. Your confidence allowed us to share something very special.

You all have made it a joy to be called...

"DOCTOR."

Table of Contents

Introduction i

Chapter 1—Keeping the Pipes Open 1

Chapter 2—Hypertension 12

Chapter 3—Medications 18

Chapter 4—Bad Stuff From Grilling 24

Chapter 5—Diabetes Mellitus; Metabolic Syndrome 27

Chapter 6—Obesity; Inflammation 42

Chapter 7—The Laboratory Tests and What They Mean 47

Chapter 8—Smoking: The Evils Thereof 57

Chapter 9—Diet; That Much; Rewards; Glycemic Index 61

Chapter 10—Exercise 82

Chapter 11—The Yearly Physical 88

Chapter 12—Putting It All Together 91

References 99

Introduction—Part 1

This is a story of how our bodies work as seen through many years of taking care of people's health problems. I am a family practice doctor with 40 years of experience in the field.

My past experience includes five years of teaching math and science along with five years of working in the medical laboratories of military hospitals and in Indiana University Medical Center. My experience as a Flight Examiner for the Federal Aviation Administration has helped to keep me up to date with the changes that are happening daily in medicine.

My hospital experience has included handling both strokes and heart attacks in the emergency room and at the bedside.

I have seen and continue to see people making horrible mistakes in their healthcare every day, and I hope to let you know some of the things that I believe do work and some that do not work in preventing bad things from happening to you.

This book is dedicated to the PREVENTION of problems that are very serious to your health.

It is my fervent hope that if you read my book you will be convinced that it is time to make some changes in YOUR life.

Thank you for your interest in my book.

Even as I partially collapsed onto the arm of the sofa, I still did not comprehend that I had suffered a stroke affecting my left leg. I continued to believe that I must have been "sitting wrong" on the sofa. When my denial finally ended and I checked into a hospital, I continued to be amazed that a physician with my experience in strokes and heart attacks would not have pressed the "action button" a lot earlier than I did. It is very easy now to see why folks do not get to their doctors sooner than they do in their time of need.

Fortunately, the use of my leg returned after a few hours, as did the use of my left arm, following a similar episode with my arm a few months later.

During these times of stress, I underwent a very thorough medical checkup and was found to be "healthy." My blood pressure was in the "normal" range as was my weight, cholesterol tests, blood sugar, etc.

But yet the MRI of my brain did show some mild damage still remaining. Fortunately, the areas were small. My patients never knew that I had had a problem because I had only lost a week of work on each occasion.

I was very aware of the problems that lead to strokes such as I had suffered and realized that even though the testing that was done on me was "normal" they were NOT normal at all.

The conditions in my body were such that the arterial blockages had happened.

This meant that I needed to make some changes in my life and do it very quickly to prevent further problems.

So, heeding the advice that I have given to my patients over so many years, I cut back on my work. I stopped delivering babies, stopped emergency room work, cut back on my hours in the office, AND began a close inspection of my body.

I quickly came to the conclusion that NORMAL, according to the experts, is sometimes not good enough to prevent the type of problems that my patients and myself were experiencing.

Over the past several years, health information has been changing and the understanding of how "bad things" happen have been expanding so rapidly that I needed more time to devote to researching and disseminating the knowledge that I have accumulated in trying to prevent these horrendous blockages from happening.

Therefore, I closed my office, but have kept all the information lines open, so that I could spend the time needed to put together this book. Some of my patients will undoubtedly see themselves on these pages. They will, in their minds, visualize me wagging my finger at them to get them to change their ways. I want them to know that I dearly love them all, but do continue my advice:

"SHAPE UP!"

I must admit that the urgency to get this into print is furthered by my continuing to observe cars flocking into the fast-food places for BREAKFAST! Talk about suicidal behavior! It drives me crazy to see this happening after all we have learned about how the body works and how it can also fall apart. This only increases my desire to get my message out. The doctors already know the message. Many patients apparently have not been told or are not listening.

I have been amazed at how many of my patients were lacking in the basic skills of being "heart healthy." Over the years I have developed "quickie lectures" for many of the items that I deemed really important. I feel that the patients that I dealt with were very grateful for this and did put that information to good use.

This book represents a series of those talks and discussions that I have had with my patients in attempting to solve their health problems. It is also aimed towards trying to prevent health problems in the first place. Many of my patients have had bad habits that the patients KNEW were bad habits, but the patients had just never been pushed to change them. I have taken it onto myself to be the "pusher." Get angry with me if you want.

Many have. I would rather that happen than see a healthy person suddenly, out of the blue, become a very unhealthy person.

One of the common scenarios that I have encountered is this: a 50-year-old person feels fine. He is 25 pounds overweight and eats pretty much what he feels like. He doesn't exercise much and sees a doctor only when he has a cold or a pain. Checkups are not deemed to be necessary so long as he is feeling well. Then, he has a heart attack. If he comes out of that, quite often with heart damage, he goes on to a rigorous schedule of cardiac rehabilitation, dietary changes, weight loss, and close follow-up with his physician. These folks often do remarkably well after they get into their rehabilitation programs. They lose weight, get their cholesterol levels in good shape, and often walk five miles three times a week on the treadmill.

In my practice this was what USUALLY happened, not what happened OCCASIONALLY.

This is WRONG. This should be reversed. The weight loss, changed lifestyle, exercise, and dietary restrictions should come BEFORE the damage to the heart happens.

One goal of this book is to convince you, the reader, that PREVENTION is most important and so much more efficient than trying to REPAIR the damage once it has occurred.

It has been known since the Korean War that young teenage soldiers, apparently healthy, when autopsied after a death caused by injury, were found to have the changes present of coronary artery disease. These soldiers had been completely without symptoms of any heart disease. Since those findings were published, many teenagers and young adults have been autopsied after accidental deaths. The same "fatty streaks" have been found in their arteries!

These fatty streaks that are found are the first signs of atherosclerosis. If you think you are immune, how about this little gem: in one autopsy study of almost three thousand men and women aged 15 to 34 years ALL OF THEM had fatty streaks in their aortas!

This shows that it was just a matter of time before these people would have had the problems associated with atherosclerosis (blocking of the arteries) and coronary artery disease if something wasn't done to prevent this cascade from happening.

There must be a really large bunch of people who are just walking time bombs, with heart attacks lurking in their future. Most of them feel "fine" and are blissfully ignorant of what awaits them.

Over the years, in caring for my patients, I have attempted to find the problems that lead to a heart attack and to correct these problems before the heart attack happens. When I have found blocked arteries and have successfully aborted a heart attack, the patient is always very surprised; for most of these patients have had NO symptoms. Quite often they really object to getting testing because they feel so well. Some of those people that are found to have problems have gone on to have corrective procedures. They often get one of the following procedures: 1) Angioplasty, which entails opening the arteries up with a catheter and balloon, maybe with a stent, to better keep the artery open. 2) Cardiac bypass graft, which entails taking an artery from somewhere, like a leg, placing it into a site that is short of circulation because of a blocked artery, and 3) Some are treated medically.

This Medical Management consists of most of the things that I am going to be advising you to do BEFORE you get to that point. That is what this book is about.

The decision concerning which of the above-listed procedures is chosen is dependent upon the type of problem and the age and health of the patient.

I will discuss how the lipoprotein called LDL enters into this picture and what to do about this nasty.

Another thing to keep in mind is the fact that in one out of every ten myocardial infarctions the FIRST symptom is SUDDEN DEATH.

So, please explore with me some of the workings of this body of yours and see what we can do to make YOUR future possibly more comfortable and less incapacitated by the injuries that might happen which are associated with that nasty and dangerous LDL.

Chapter 1—Keeping the Pipes Open

I have never taken any exercise except when sleeping or resting.

Mark Twain

It used to be thought that "hardening of the arteries" was like having a cement block in the arteries. You lived or died according to how much limitation there was of the blood flow to your vital organs. Then, one of the most remarkable findings ever to come out of medicine happened. Let me tell you about it.

Some years ago a man had severe heart disease to such an extent that he was not able to have the usual bypass graft of arteries to the heart to give the heart a fresh blood supply. For most people in this circumstance, it would have meant that he would have been doomed to a life of severe disability and finally death. This did not happen to this gentleman. His very wise physician prescribed a VERY low-fat diet. I mean this diet was BAD!

One year later his coronary angiograms (X-rays showing arterial circulation using dye injection in the arteries) were free of the clogging particles (plaques) that had caused the problem!

This shook up the medical world! This study showed conclusively that the arteries are in a continual state of change. Those are not hard rocks in there. And if the arteries are "hard," they may become "softer" with treatment. They are changing all the time! That means that if your arteries have some of these changes, with some modification in your lifestyle that I am going to suggest, these changes can actually improve, and in very short order!

Note: Most of the results gotten with lipid lowering are not as dramatic as are the results that are mentioned above. It is not unusual to get results at six months, but the results in benefit are greater than one would predict by what is observed in the shrinkage of the plaques. Coronary angiograms have shown the lumen (inside diameter) increasing at three years after the start of statin therapy.

The Endothelium

The endothelium is the lining of all of our blood vessels. This includes the microscopic-sized vessels.

When we discuss coronary artery disease we must discuss this lining of our arteries. It is one of the most remarkable organs in this remarkable body of ours. It is there to help us to stay healthy. It does a pretty good job of doing that as long as we don't screw up and prevent it from doing its job. When the endothelium, for one reason or another, isn't doing its job, the condition is called "endothelial dysfunction."

The endothelium is the gatekeeper for what happens inside the artery walls. It is supposed to keep the good stuff in and the bad stuff out. This ability to modify what can go in and out is called "permeability." This permeability can be really messed up and allow fatty plaques to form in the arteries by way of a number of different things happening. You can already guess what they are.

Some of the main problems that cause the endothelium not to work effectively are: atherosclerosis (hardening of the arteries), smoking, hyperlipidemia (high cholesterol-type substances), family history of premature coronary artery disease, diabetes, heart failure, and angina pectoris with normal coronary arteries (syndrome x).

Unfortunately, advancing age also cuts down on the endothelium's ability to do its job.

What a pity!

There are a few surprises here, too.

There are tests that can show the arteries actually changing as various conditions are imposed on them. These tests are not available for clinical use but give us an idea, research-wise, of what things can cause arterial change. It was found, using these tests, that a brief period of mental stress like you and I have a dozen times a day can prevent the endothelium from doing its job! Even just recalling in your mind something that upset you in the past can do it. Type-A personalities take note.

It has been shown that endothelial dysfunction is the first step in the formation of atherosclerosis.

Because the endothelium is not able to do its job properly, maybe for one of the above-listed reasons, it becomes "permeable" (opened to passage) to substances that ordinarily cannot get into the blood vessel wall. When the endothelium is injured in one way or another, LDL can pass through the wall, and with a process called "oxidation," it becomes more of a threat. This allows other cells to enter and join the crowd. Among these cells are "foam cells" and macrophages (infection fighters) that are responding to the body's alarm that something is not going well.

Doesn't "foam cell" have an ominous sound to it?

It certainly does not bode well for a foam cell's owner that it is there. Under the microscope it looks like "foam" inside the cell. It has little pockets of stuff crammed into it that most cells don't have.

And, what do you think is in those pockets?

You probably have already guessed.

These cells are loaded with fat, cholesterol, in fact.

Because the cell is loaded with cholesterol, it often dies. The products of the cell's death cause a release of various chemicals that call up more cells to join the battle.

And this is what really makes the stuff hit the fan because this mass is so unstable. As the various types of cells bunch up in the artery wall, you have this mass of soft spongy material making up part of it. There is no way that this mess will act predictably when under pressure. Because of this basic instability in the plaque that has formed, this mass can break apart and cause problems at any time. When it breaks apart, the pieces can go into the bloodstream and cause clogging and the shutting off of blood flow on down the line. This may end up causing a myocardial infarction if it shuts off the blood supply sufficiently. Or, the spot where the plaque broke apart can act as a nidus (spot for a larger clump of cells to form) continuing to put the poor vessel, and you, at risk.

Once it's there, it can be gotten rid of, but I'm sure that you agree that it would be much more satisfactory in this case not to let it be formed in the first place.

That's the purpose of this whole book.

As you can see above, the well-being of the endothelium is the key to having healthy blood vessels. So let's discuss this a bit more. Stick with me.

If the endothelium receives an insult and the condition of "endothelial dysfunction" happens, the permeability changes and allows LDL into the blood vessel wall that the endothelium is lining. The endothelium is exquisitely sensitive to change when challenged by the LDL-type fats. The LDL goes through a process of oxidation that makes it a more dangerous and deadly material. The first changes that happen are that the blood vessels lose some of their elasticity. This automatically brings about an increase in blood pressure as, with each heartbeat, the stiff vessel transmits this increased pressure on down the line instead of absorbing it by enlarging in diameter temporarily. The next thing one sees as the changes continue to happen are "fatty streaks" forming in the blood vessel walls. These changes are seen as thickening of the intima (endothelium) with accompanying lipid (fat) deposits both inside and outside the cells. So we really want to prevent this chain of events from coming about. This means we must prevent or correct the endothelial dysfunction that was behind all of this in the first place.

Still with me?

Hang in there.

Some things that have been found to reverse the Endothelial Dysfunction once it's there are: 1) Stop cigarette smoking, 2) Take L-Arginine, 3) Fix elevated lipids in the blood, 4) Use Estrogen replacement, 5) Use Antioxidants, and 6) Use ACE Inhibitors.

Let's look at these things.

Stopping smoking is a no-brainer. Right? From all the things previously discussed, it becomes rather obvious that this HAS to happen. The injury to this marvelous endothelium is certain and severe. But it is reversible. The solution: If you are a smoker, stop smoking! If you are not a smoker, good for you!

L-Arginine

This is an amino acid that is present in all forms of life. It is made by the organism. It is a "precursor" in the formation of nitric oxide. This means that as the body goes through its various steps to produce nitric oxide L-Arginine is one of the substances that is formed before getting to nitric oxide. Nitric oxide (NO) is a great vessel dilator. It actually allows more blood to flow through any given blood vessel. It is known to prevent constriction of blood vessels. As a result it makes sense that it would be of help in preventing or treating atherosclerosis, hypertension, hyperlipidemia, and angina pectoris.

L-Arginine has been found not only to improve endothelium-dependent dilation of a blood vessel but also reduces the monocyte adhesion (blood cells sticking together to make a clump) to endothelial cells in young men with coronary artery disease.

L-Arginine comes from both animal and plant protein. Soy protein and other plant proteins are richer in it than animal sources. The body's need for it increases in periods of stress such as infection, trauma and burns.

There have been some claims that it might be a "fat burner" and might help one to lose weight, but so far those claims have not been substantiated.

Its role in erectile dysfunction is looked upon as "promising." If one looks at the advertisements, one would think that it had been proven beyond the shadow of a doubt that it helps to correct erectile dysfunction.

Correcting Lipids

Correcting the lipids is the subject of most of this book. It is sometimes not easy, but it can be remarkably rapid. The great thing is that endothelial dysfunction is reversible, and we are not necessarily stuck with the problem forever.

Lipid values that are not as desirable as what we would like can be corrected, so don't get discouraged along the way.

Estrogen Replacement

Many of us who have been in medicine for a while would swear that post-menopausal women lived longer and with a better quality of life when they were taking estrogen. Their skins remained younger looking and softer than those who did not receive hormone replacement. The cardiac status of the women on estrogen seemed improved over those not on estrogen. So, when the Women's Health Initiative came along, it personally CRUSHED me. That study suggested that there was an INCREASED risk of coronary disease in those ladies who were taking hormone replacement. The study was stopped to prevent any harm from befalling those women who were taking part in the study.

The Women's Heath Initiative was a long-term study that followed thousands of women. The study compared the health problems of those women who were taking hormone replacement with those who were not.

When those results were published, I reluctantly advised my ladies who were taking estrogen to stop that medication until more was known about the side effects. Now, with more time for analyzing the results, it appears that maybe the estrogen isn't so bad, but the estrogen-progesterone combination has continued to be a "forbidden."

Actually, when looking at estrogen's beneficial effect on the endothelial function, it appears that estrogen might still be a valuable medication for the post-menopausal woman. We doctors are still quaking from the results of that WHI study and want to be darned sure about the drug's safety before placing our women back on them.

It is now known that progesterone nullifies any benefit that estrogen has on the endothelium. (Explanation: Ladies who still have a uterus cannot take estrogen alone, but must have it combined with a drug called progesterone because of a very definite increased risk of uterine cancer when estrogen is used alone. Ladies without a uterus can take the estrogen by itself.)

There was a study prior to the WHI called the Nurses Health Study that did show a 40-50% reduction in the number of heart attacks among those women who were taking estrogen.

The discussions go on.

Antioxidants

I take mine every day. Do you take yours?

Remember earlier I said that LDL underwent this "oxidation" process that made it a more deadly molecule to the body? O.K. Here we have an antioxidant (read that as anti-oxidation medication) and that is what they do. Or what they are supposed to do.

There is another term that we need to deal with here, so hang on a bit longer.

That is the "Free Radical."

Every day our bodies are being bombarded with things that can injure it. These can create "free radicals." The damage might come from the sun's rays that cause damage to a skin cell so that, if nothing stops the process, it might go on to become a skin cancer. The same goes for the cells in the colon that have been damaged by the carcinogens in something that we ate (read that as "grilled meat," see "Bad Stuff From Grilling" chapter) that could go on to become a colon cancer. Our own cells, during their divisions, repairing, and dying, often create imperfections. These can undergo this "oxidation" which makes them more of a problem.

We hope that by getting antioxidants every day we can prevent some of these oxidations from happening or nullify them if they do happen.

The commercial companies certainly know that we are in the market for these. You see their advertising daily—the green tea, grape juice, and wine, to name a few. Of course we have the pill that we can take daily just to be sure that we are getting enough antioxidants.

I have been in this business long enough to see a lot of swings in thinking on how much benefit there is from taking antioxidants. There was a time that vitamin E, an antioxidant, was thought to prevent heart failure. You don't see that discussed anymore, but looking at its beneficial action on the endothelium, maybe there WAS something to that theory.

There was an "aspirin and antioxidant" study many years ago. This study has since saved a bunch of lives and continues to save them daily. That study showed two things: 1) An aspirin a day could help prevent a myocardial infarction, and 2) An antioxidant a day could reduce the incidence of colon cancer.

Since that study came out, I haven't missed my low-dose aspirin or my antioxidant pill and have advised my patients to do the same.

A word of warning just came out in 2005. You CAN get too much of a good thing. It seems that when you get too many antioxidants on board, they may work in a way opposite to what they are supposed to work.

How much is too much? No one knows.

Keep an eye on your newspapers to see how this shakes out. It may well be that we are seeing another swing away from antioxidants. At present I believe it is wise to stay away from large doses of ANY vitamin. Whenever possible, get your vitamins from your good healthful foods.

Moderation has worked over the centuries. I think that it is still good advice.

BE KIND TO YOUR ENDOTHELIUM.

(That would make a nice saying for a tee shirt.)

Now, let's get down to the nitty-gritty of this thing and talk about what these substances are that give us so much grief. Then we will go on to figure out what we can do about them.

There are actually at least three different ways that a coronary artery can be a problem to its owner.

An artery can go into "spasm" which can be brought on by many different things. See the chapter on "Smoking" for more on that particular cause. It has also been shown that both elevated levels of insulin and high levels of fats in the blood can cause this spasm.

A second way that an artery can be a problem to its owner is where a "plaque" sits in the artery. This is what shows up on the studies as a certain percent "blockage" of the artery. These plaques become symptomatic when they obstruct about 70% to 80% of the artery opening. This is what causes "angina" in a heart patient.

When the patient exercises, the blockage may be enough that the area of the heart to which the artery is going gets in trouble because of not having enough oxygen delivered to take care of its needs during that exercise. Chest pain, called "angina pectoris," may result. The well-known drug nitroglycerin may dilate the artery enough that the angina is relieved. That does not solve the problem. If the area of the heart is REALLY in trouble, the lack of oxygen may result in injury to the heart. We call this a "myocardial infarction" (heart attack).

The third problem that can happen in an artery is more sneaky and difficult to detect. Here a bunch of fatty substance (LDL) layers are out under the inner lining of the artery in sort of a glob. This area becomes thickened and may set up an inflammation to which cells of the body respond in an attempt to repair the damage. As a result the weakened wall of the artery may rupture into the interior of the artery causing an obstruction to blood flow that mimics the obstruction detailed above. This can have the same devastating results, namely myocardial infarction. Actually the death and disability rate is higher for this third type than the obviously obstructed type.

There are many factors involved in why a plaque ruptures. They are too involved to describe here. Certainly inflammation with its influence on the cells to clump together is present in all plaques.

How do you know if you have this type of problem?

This non-obstructive type generally does not show up on standard testing. I instruct my patients to assume that if their cholesterol panel is way out of whack that they do have one or both of the above-listed types of problems, just not enough to cause symptoms yet. They should also assume that as their lipid panel improves, as they do all the great things that their friendly doctor has instructed them to do, that the fatty deposits of both kinds will be dissolving away. Remember that HDL has the ability to remove LDL fat particles, so let's get that HDL up there! For details see "The Laboratory Tests and What They Mean."

When we start to discuss what things come into play in keeping the pipes open, or to open the clogged ones, high on the list has to be diet. This supplies the raw materials that our bodies have to use as building blocks. After all, the body has to use them; that's all there is. So, if one constructed a building using faulty or poor quality materials, the building is certainly going to suffer and will not be a very good building. The same goes for our bodies. We know that certain materials are necessary for a healthy body. The government approves a "food pyramid" which contains the proteins, carbohydrates, etc. that make up the required ingredients. The problem is that within each of the food types there are some good foods and some not so good. You should check out the pyramid and use this book in helping you to make good decisions on how to modify the pyramid's suggestions.

We will be emphasizing the role that obesity plays in heart disease. *USA Today* in 2005 reported from the journal *Health Affairs* about obesity-tied healthcare. They reported a ten-fold rise in costs of healthcare for obese individuals as compared to the non-obese between 1987 and 2002, the latest figures available. They report, "The growth in obesity has fueled a dramatic increase in the amount spent in treating diabetes, heart disease, high cholesterol, and other weight-related illnesses." They further reported, "Overall, employers and privately-insured spent $36.5 billion on obesity-related illnesses in 2002, up from $3.6 billion in 1987."

Just how early in life do we see coronary disease?

When autopsies were done on healthy soldiers that were killed in the Korean War, it was found that these "healthy" teens and early-twenties males already had coronary artery disease!

Actually, cardiovascular disease will affect the MAJORITY of individuals by age 60.

At this point we have to mention a study that has been a huge help to us in knowing and understanding what works and what doesn't work in our healthcare. It was called the Framingham Heart Study; 7,733 people of Framingham, Massachusetts, allowed themselves to be tested and followed over many years. The investigators came up with all sorts of great facts about what happens to people that were just not known before that time. We should be forever grateful to those people for allowing themselves to be the subjects of this huge investigation. Among the things that were found out is the fact that, starting with people free of heart disease, the lifetime risk at age 40 for men was 49 percent and for women it was 32 percent. Even for people who were free of heart disease at age 70, their risk was still there with 35 percent for men and 24 percent for women. This, of course, is disastrous for the people involved, because most of the people with this disease die of the disease. It is also very expensive for society to have this happening.

In the Interheart Study in Europe, it was found that there were nine potentially modifiable factors that accounted for population-attributable risk of a first heart attack. These included being a smoker, having or not having high blood pressure, being a diabetic or not being a diabetic, being obese in the abdominal region as compared to other regions, psychosocial factors, regular alcohol consumption (a little is good every day. I will say more about that later), daily consumption of fruits and vegetables, and getting exercise daily.

Just think about that for a bit.

Nine out of ten heart attacks might have been prevented with the modification of those nine risk factors!

I think that each of us at this point really needs to sit back and study this, because it really doesn't seem like an overwhelming task to accomplish.

It is interesting to note that weight enters into hypertension, abdominal obesity, and diabetes. What a nice place to begin the attack.

Over the past twenty years, about one million Americans have died of cardiovascular disease EVERY year in the US. About 700,000 people have strokes each year in the US. In general, when you find hardening of the arteries with the associated changes in one part of the body, these changes are usually present throughout the entire body. For instance, if a person had a heart attack because the vessels of the heart were affected, probably this person is also at increased risk of stroke, leg pain when walking, and aortic aneurysm.

That doesn't seem fair, does it?

I can't think of a better reason to put a lot of emphasis on PREVENTION, because the risks are so great when things get out of hand.

Chapter 2—Hypertension

He who takes medicine and neglects diet wastes the skill of his doctors.

Chinese Proverb

Blood pressure has long been known to be a factor in the prevention of heart attacks and strokes. You can imagine that if your blood pressure is elevated your arteries are going to be pounded all day and all night by this increased pressure. This is bound to make some changes in the vessels and thus to the organs that the vessels supply. Each year the "powers that be" lower what is thought to be "normal" blood pressure just as they have lowered the values that are "normal" for blood sugar, the cholesterol panel values, etc., etc. They do this because they find that blood pressures that were previously called "normal" caused complications, some of them being severe.

It is very important for you to know what your blood pressure is. If you know what it is and it is not where you want it, you should do something about it. Some of the BP ranges found at the pharmacies, etc., may be labeled as "normal," but if they do not fall in line with the following, they need to be improved.

What should your BP be? It is becoming more difficult each year to be "normal." The latest classifications at the time of this printing are:

Optimal	115/75 or less
Normal	120/80 or less
Prehypertension	139/89 or less
Stage 1 Hypertension	159/99 or less
Stage 2 Hypertension	160/100 or above

Do not be satisfied until the top number (hereafter called "systolic") is in the 120s, but 130s is "not bad" and the bottom number ("diastolic") is in the 60s, but 70s is "not bad."

In your particular case you may not be able to reach it, but those more desirable numbers should be your "goal."

You should have a blood pressure monitoring device at home so that you can check the pressure at whatever interval you and your physician deem necessary. If you do not have a monitor, you should get one. These pressure devices are easy to use and for the most part are accurate when they are used as directed. You should not feel uneasy about using one at home.

If your blood pressure is doing well, checking it once a month may be all that is needed. If the pressure hasn't been behaving too well, you may need to check it daily to see what the problem is.

Everyone's blood pressure drops at night so that is not a good time to do your checking. You need to know what your blood pressure is doing during the day when you are up and active. You should take several pressures in a row, just as your doctor may be doing. You will usually find that the first one is the highest, so that if that set of numbers is "just dandy" there is no need to take more. But if it is not so great, then you should take two additional readings at intervals of three minutes. If the blood pressure isn't down by that time, you should so note and then see if there is a trend on a day-to-day basis. If you cannot fix the problem, you should see your friendly physician.

Just a few notes about blood pressure monitoring. I have had people wonder about our office readings because we never seem to get the same reading two times in a row. This is because the blood pressure is changing CONSTANTLY! The body has a continuously operating set of checks and balances. Let's just examine what happens when we get up from a chair to get something. Because we have changed our position, some blood will leave the upper body and drop into the legs. To counteract that drop, the muscles in the legs must contract and try to push the blood back up. If the person's system isn't working very well, for example, when one has been in bed for a week because of an illness, the person may become lightheaded as the blood leaves the brain because of the position change. The leg muscles were out of practice. This person needs to sit back down. Next time the person needs to get up more slowly and allow the body a bit more time to make that adjustment. The person who is physically fit will not have that happen because the muscles of the legs are more than able to squeeze down and not allow the brain to get shortchanged.

A good example of this happening comes in observing the astronauts as they return to earth after being in space in a weightless condition. They do their best while in space to keep their bodies in good shape, but most of them have a bit of trouble walking without getting lightheaded and dizzy, as the process outlined above happens.

So you may find that your blood pressure is a little high or a little low when getting up from a chair. The body will do what it needs to do in order to keep the brain supplied with an adequate amount of blood.

Likewise, when we are sleeping, the body's demands are few, and hopefully the blood pressure will be at its lowest.

Some of the highest blood pressures that I have seen have been in truck drivers. Bless their hearts. They have to stay awake over the many hours on the road, and often take drugs to help them stay awake. Their most popular drug is caffeine, with many of my drivers drinking a pot or two of coffee a day. This fires up their systems, including their blood pressures. It is not unusual to find blood pressures of 220/110! I am amazed that the drivers' bodies can handle pressures like these and not have very serious problems. And, I am sure, over a period of time, this HAS to be damaging their organ systems. When I examine these gentlemen for their commercial driving license and find this kind of pressure, they do not pass the exam. I then advise them to stop all coffee and see me in 48 hours. Quite often their pressures are perfectly normal after that length of time free of caffeine. At that time I try to warn them of the risks that they are taking with those elevated blood pressures. They generally do get their licenses renewed. Hopefully they will change their ways after that experience. I can only hope that my warnings have made a difference in their lives.

As you are trying out your new blood pressure apparatus, you will notice that on some days your blood pressure is definitely higher than on other days. It is a good idea to try to figure out why there is a difference from day to day. Did you have an argument with your tax consultant? Did you just finish paying for a tank full of gas? Did you just get a promotion?

Emotions figure into this business of blood pressure. However, so do some other things. High on the list is salt intake. By now you should know that you should be selecting foods and drinks that are low in sodium. Sometimes, however, you are stuck with having to eat an increased salt load. Almost all of the commercially prepared microwave meals are really loaded with salt. If you happen to eat one, or have some other salty food, you will surely find that your blood pressure is a little higher on the next day. That salt (sodium) made your body retain water, which in turn made your blood pressure rise. This is because of the increased volume in your circulatory system. As you drink water, the salt is gotten rid of through the urine, and the blood pressure should return to normal.

We should touch on a term that you may hear, and a condition that you might have. That is the "White Coat Syndrome." This is the condition wherein your blood pressure goes up when you get in the doctor's office. It is very common. Some of my patients that have known me all of their lives (I delivered them.) have told me that they can feel their blood pressure rise when they enter my office…and I don't wear a white coat. If your blood pressure monitor is showing lower blood pressures than those that your physician is getting, you should carefully document those blood pressures and try to convince all concerned that this is happening. Thus you may avoid being placed on medications that may do you harm.

Being tired can make your blood pressure rise. The hospital intern finishing up his 12-hour shift will probably have an elevated blood pressure. Of course, the coffee that was consumed during that time does not help either.

People wonder which number, the systolic (upper) or the diastolic (lower), is the more important of the two. Of course they are both important because they reflect the pounding that your arteries are taking with each beat of your heart. It is now known, from studies of people with kidney failure as a result of hypertension, that elevation of the systolic blood pressure brings about kidney failure earlier than does elevation of the diastolic blood pressure.

There was a fairly recent study done with almost 9,000 people that showed what they called "prehypertension" (130-139/85-89) was associated with an increased risk of cardiovascular disease, stroke, and heart failure. I would imagine that, because of these findings, this range of blood pressures will be added to those that define "hypertension."

I have had many patients who really didn't see what all the fuss was about when their blood pressures were less than ideal.

Just what DOES happen when uncontrolled hypertension extends over a long period time? Well, I can tell you it's not pretty!

When the blood vessels are being pounded by increased pressures, the normal cellular structure of the blood vessels starts to change. We call this process "remodeling." As the high pressures continue, the heart must enlarge to continue to do the work of supplying blood to the body. There comes a point where the heart muscle will not be able to enlarge anymore.

At this point the heart can no longer handle the load imposed on it, and as a result there may be fluids retained by the body. We call this fluid "edema." At this point the life expectancy of the individual has really decreased. Even with all of our great medications to treat this "heart failure," the patient's future course is rather dismal. You really never want this to happen to you or to your loved ones.

The moral: normalize your blood pressure.

In fact, hypertension at age 50 has been found to shorten the lifespan of both men and women by five years compared with 50-year-olds who had normal blood pressure. The causes of death included cardiovascular disease, myocardial infarction, and stroke.

And, going on to the congestive heart failure stage, research has shown that the incidence of heart failure can be cut in half simply by controlling the blood pressure!

Medicare spends more dollars on the diagnosis and treatment of heart failure than on any other disease entity.

Now, we come back to the awful term "obesity." Research is going on continually and, almost on a daily basis, new findings are being reported. The American Heart Association reports research showing that when young healthy adults gain weight (fat) their arteries get stiffer which leads to higher blood pressures. The good news is that this process is reversible. So, as you lose weight the arteries will lose some of their stiffness. This should allow the blood pressure to decrease. By the way, this process is also found in children in their teens!

I have always known that when my patients lose weight their blood pressure does go down, but I always figured that it was the body's response to carrying around a lesser load. So maybe both the decreased load and the lessened stiffness of the arteries are at work here.

Chapter 3—Medications

*Half the modern drugs could well be thrown out the window,
except that the birds might eat them.*

Martin H. Fisher

Well, we sure don't want to take medicines that are not necessary.

The following is a partial list of drugs that are used to help keep
the pipes open. The side-effect profile, drug interactions, etc., are
not shown. Your doctor should be consulted before taking any of
them.

Aspirin

This is some kind of medication! You have been bombarded with
information about this drug. It is looked down on by a lot of
people because it is so cheap. But, let me tell you, if it were
discovered today in our drug climate, it would be darned
expensive because it has so many great properties. But, like the
advertising says, "It is not for everyone."

First of all, if you have some sort of known bleeding disorder, you
would certainly need your doctor's input on whether or not you
should take it. If you have had a bleeding ulcer, you would
certainly need your doctor's advice. If you take NSAIDS (non-
steroidal anti-inflammatory drugs), there is an increased incidence
of gastrointestinal bleed, and that would warrant more caution in
taking low-dose aspirin. Low-dose aspirin, 81 mgm, is generally
used because it has been found that the good preventative effects
on the blood vessels are as good with low dose as they are with the
higher doses, and the risk of complication is much less (mostly
bleeding and irritation). Keep tuned in, because this
recommendation may change in the next several years.

One of aspirin's properties is that it cuts down on platelet aggregation (clumping together). The platelets are necessary for the clot formation that prevents us from bleeding to death with minor, or not so minor, injuries. But platelets can also be a problem in arteries when there is inflammation or other injury. For example, if there is a plaque in an artery which produces a narrowing, the platelets may clump up, set off a chain reaction of various cells coming into the region, and subsequently cause a blockage of the artery.

A report from the Archives of Neurology suggests that if you are taking aspirin regularly and you should suddenly stop taking it, you may be at INCREASED risk of heart attack or stroke. So, if you are going to take aspirin as a preventer of heart attack and stroke, you should be a good pill-taker and not miss doses or discontinue the medication without consulting your doctor.

We know that inflammation plays a huge role in heart disease, along with other diseases. It is thought that aspirin reduces the body's ability to produce a hormone-like substance called "prostaglandin." Thus, the aspirin decreases pain, is thought to reduce inflammation, and decreases platelet aggregation. This is quite a bunch of really good things out of that little pill.

For the most part, I advise people to start an 81-mgm tablet daily at age 40. This, of course, should be discussed with your doctor. I am continually amazed, however, as I talk to the general public, how many people have not taken advantage of this great preventer of BIG problems. Unless you have some problem that keeps you from it, be sure YOU take advantage of it. EVERY DAY.

When you take your one aspirin a day, you will note that you bruise more easily. Women, especially, hate this bruising because it is so unsightly. It is very difficult to keep women from discontinuing aspirin. This bruising should be looked upon as proof that the medication is working. After all, we are trying to prevent clot buildup in our arteries. The bruising with minor trauma is proof that the aspirin is doing what it is supposed to do. If you have bruising without trauma, be sure to check with your doctor.

I have people ask about aspirin risk in case of an accident or a severe cut where bleeding is a real problem. I agree that having this drug on board is going to increase the bleeding risk, so each person must make that decision on their own. They must decide which risk is greater, heart disease or bleeding from trauma.

With all this said, it is not easy to keep a lot of my patients taking this drug. Many revert back to taking it only occasionally for minor aches and pains. They have forgotten my lecture!

How dare they!

The Statins

The battle continues today about how to use the statins. They work by blocking an enzyme in the liver that the liver needs to produce cholesterol. The statins do bring down total cholesterol, raise that good HDL, lower the triglycerides, and decrease that nasty LDL. That is a lot to ask of a single drug! It has been a remarkable drug in helping to combat the Killer LDL. There is still a fear among some investigators and doctors that the statins may be harmful. On the other hand, some physicians think that they are safe enough and valuable enough that they ought to be sold over-the-counter.

I believe that they should remain as prescription drugs. There are a couple of very serious problems that are possible while taking the statins that make me continue to drag my feet on loosening the reins on these drugs. One is liver damage.

All of the statins that are currently on the market have to have liver testing done at various intervals after being started. This testing has to be continued for as long as the drugs are taken. It is very rare to have a liver blood test that is elevated enough that the drug has to be discontinued, but damage to the liver is something that you certainly would NOT want to miss. Unfortunately, early damage can only be detected through blood testing.

The other serious problem is one affecting the muscles. There is a very severe illness called "rhabdomyalysis" in which the muscles are severely damaged. This is a condition that is rare but possible. It seems that when the muscle is damaged the products of the breakdown are really toxic to the kidneys. Myoglobin is one of the products. It is released into the bloodstream and then is filtered through the kidneys. Under certain circumstances it can cause "acute tubular necrosis" to the kidney. In this condition the tubules in the kidneys are actually destroyed and one can actually see parts of this debris in the urine under the microscope. This necrosis can also go on to cause kidney failure in which case the person actually has to go onto dialysis in order to survive.

Many people have less severe muscle aches and pains when they take these drugs. It is important to discuss this with your physician if you should experience any muscle pains after starting the statins. There are blood tests that can be done to differentiate the serious from the not so serious, if your doctor feels the need to do them after listening to your story.

The trend in using statins has been to go "all out" and to get the total cholesterol and LDL as low as we can. There has been benefit shown in each trial as the values were pushed lower.

At the present time this is the group of statins that are available: Atorvastatin (Lipitor), Fluvastatin (Lescol), Lovastatin (Mevacor), Pravastatin (Pravachol), Rosuvastatin (Crestor), and Simvastatin (Zocor).

Most of the experts in the field agree that all of these drugs work. The companies that make them can cite 101 reasons why their drug is superior to all of the others. And, indeed, there are differences, but most doctors are comfortable with using the cheaper generic drugs that the insurance companies will cover.

There have been many studies that show that the calcium-volume scores of the heart actually decrease after a minimum of 12 months of statin therapy. This means that if the person has calcium in the arteries that the calcium became measurably less after 12 months on medication. In other studies there has been shown increases in the inside diameter of affected arteries after two and four years of statin therapy. Who says that these are hard rocks in the arteries that can't be changed?

Ezetimibe (Zetia)

This is a relatively recent addition to the drugs that work on the cholesterol problem. This drug works in the bowel to prevent reabsorption of the cholesterol products. Since the statins work in the liver, you get sort of a one-two punch when you use these drugs together. They have worked really well for my patients, with remarkable lowering of the LDL, both with and without the statins. They are relatively free of problems, but the company does recommend following with liver testing.

Nicotinic Acid (Niaspan)

This is a B-Vitamin drug. The mode of action of this drug is not known for sure. It is usually used when other drugs have not quite brought about the desired results or the other drugs cannot be used for one reason or another. The main side effect is "flushing" after you take it. There are some things that you can do to prevent that. Liver damage is the main complication. The company that makes it suggests that the long-acting Niaspan has fewer liver problems than the short-acting drugs, which are sold over the counter. Other sources say otherwise. Liver studies should be done to follow both formulations of the medication. This drug may affect the blood sugar, so the patient should be carefully monitored for changes.

**Colestipol (Colestid), Cholestyramine (Questran),
Cholesevelam (WelChol)**

These are Bile Acid Sequestrants used as an adjunct with diet to reduce cholesterol and LDL. They work in the bowel to bind up bile acids and prevent them from being reabsorbed. This reduces the amount of bile acids for the liver to use in producing cholesterol. They can interfere with the body's vitamin uptake, along with the uptake of some medications.

Gemfibrozil (Lopid)

Not used often. It is usually used when the triglycerides are very elevated such that there is a risk of developing pancreatitis. When used with the statins, there is a very increased risk of rhabdomyalysis happening. Close monitoring is necessary. There are other very serious side effects that limit the usefulness of this drug.

Herbals

The only herbal that I believe shows some benefit in heart protection is garlic. A report out of the University of Oxford in 1994 showed that there was evidence that garlic inhibits platelet aggregation (clumping together), increases fibrinolysis (breaks down clots), reduces blood pressure, enhances antioxidant activity, and reduces serum lipids. I have had a few patients who have done very well on garlic.

The feeling among my patients is that since herbals are "natural" they must be good. This isn't necessarily so. The main health problems associated with certain ones can be: 1) Bleeding tendencies and 2) Liver damage.

It may be that one could safely take an herbal drug that had a bleeding tendency associated with it and not get in trouble, but I have found that patients don't think in that fashion. They tend to be convinced that each of their health concerns calls for a different herbal. They tend to take these things in bunches. These people are definitely at risk of hemorrhage and liver problems when they do this. Before deciding on taking any of them, you need to check them out on the Internet, at a site that does not sell herbals. If Internet capability isn't possible, check with your local library. Be sure to inform your friendly doctor if you are taking any herbal.

Chapter 4—Bad Stuff From Grilling

Red meat is not bad for you. Now, blue-green meat, THAT'S bad for you!

Tommie Smothers

Now, we come to another problem with meats. Cancer rears its ugly head. Lots of people are not aware of the dangers associated with meat; so let me go over them with you.

When you go into the grocery store to buy meat, let's say turkey, one of your choices is going to be whether to choose roasted or smoked. You should try to stay away from cured or smoked meats. The processes that are used for preservation are harmful and do increase your risk of cancer.

When refrigeration was introduced, the incidence of colon cancer dropped dramatically as the percentage of people eating smoked or cured meats decreased. These processes introduce carcinogens into the meat so that you not only have potential problems with cholesterol products but also with potential cancer risk.

One of the American pastimes is firing up the backyard grill. The grilled food really tastes great. We really love that added smoke flavor. But again, your risks go up. However, your risks also increase with cooking your meat in the kitchen. Cooking meat can form chemicals called "heterocyclic amines" that are not present in the uncooked food. This can increase your risk of cancer in several different areas.

From the National Cancer Institute, 9/15/04:

"Research conducted by the National Cancer Institute (NCI) as well as by Japanese and European scientists indicates that heterocycyclic amines are created within muscle meats during most types of high temperature cooking.

Recent studies have further evaluated the relationship associated with methods of cooking meat and the specific types of cancer.

One study conducted by researchers from NCI's Division of cancer Epidemiology and Genetics found a link between individuals with stomach cancer and the consumption of cooked meats. The researchers assessed the diets and cooking habits of 176 people diagnosed with stomach cancer and 503 people with no evidence of cancer. The researchers found that those who ate their beef medium-well or well-done had more than three times the risk of stomach cancer compared to those who ate their beef rare or medium-rare. They also found that people who ate beef four or more times a week had more than twice the risk of developing stomach cancer compared to those consuming beef less frequently. Additional studies have shown that an increased risk of developing colorectal, pancreatic, and breast cancer is associated with high intakes of well-done, fried, or barbecued meats."

It goes on to say:

"Temperature is the most important factor in the formation of HCA's. Frying, broiling and barbecuing produce the largest amounts of HCA's because the meats are cooked at very high temperatures. One study conducted by researchers showed a three-fold increase in the content of HCA's when the cooking temperature was increased from 200 degrees to 250 degrees centigrade (392 to 482F). Oven roasting and baking are done at lower temperatures so lower levels of HCA's are likely to form. However, gravy made from meat drippings does contain substantial amounts of HCA's. Stewing, boiling, or poaching are done at or below 100 degrees centigrade (212F). Cooking at this low temperature creates negligible amounts of the chemicals. Foods cooked a long time, "well-done" instead of "medium," by other methods will also form slightly more of the chemicals."

At the present time no one knows for sure how much HCA it takes to cause a cancer. More work needs to be done on that. It is being suggested that microwaving the meats before the high-temperature preparation of the meat may cut down on the amount of HCA in the final product.

There is another problem when one prepares meat, especially in "grilling," that favorite American pastime. When fats drip onto the coals, or sizzles in the pan, bad chemicals are formed which are called Polycyclic Aromatic Hydrocarbons (PAH). What happens here is that these dangerous chemicals are formed when fats burn.

Then in the smoke they attach themselves to the meat that is being eaten. This is then ingested and the PAHs come in contact with the gastrointestinal tract where the cancers mostly occur. Evidently the time in contact with the mucosal linings is the important thing here, so that if a person has a bowel movement (BM) twice a day the contents of the colon sort of whiz right along and have less chance to cause a problem. Presumably these changes start by causing an inflammation. However, if the person only has a BM twice a week, it affords the irritant a much greater opportunity to affect the bowel lining and possibly cause a disaster.

There are grills on the market that are supposed to get around this problem by having the fat roll down grooves in the plate and be collected in a pan from which it can be discarded. I have watched these in action. What I have seen is that the grease sizzles away and very little ever gets into the pan to be discarded. This process produces, I am sure, a pretty fair amount of both PAHs and HCAs.

Back to the drawing board!

Chapter 5—Diabetes Mellitus; Metabolic Syndrome

Man seems to be a rickety sort of thing, any way you take him; a kind of British Museum of infirmities and inferiority's. He is always undergoing repairs. A machine that unreliable would have no market.

Mark Twain

There surely are a lot of diabetics out there. It is thought that there are 18 million diabetics in the US at present. Thirteen million of them are diagnosed and five million of them remain to be diagnosed. This is about 6% of the total population. There are 1.3 million getting diagnosed per year. There are another 16 million people who are classified as "prediabetic."

Diabetes is costly both to the individual and to the nation.

Some statistics concerning diabetes:

...The chief cause of blindness

...The chief cause of kidney failure

...The sixth leading cause of death

...The majority of diabetics die of heart disease.

...Three out of every four diabetics have hypertension.

...There is an increased risk of colon cancer.

...The diabetic has the SAME risk of having a heart attack as those who have had a previous heart attack.

A study called the National Health And Nutrition Examination Survey (NHANES) showed that obesity increased from 16% of the people to 30% of the people between 1960 and 2000. In that same period diabetes increased from 1.8% of the population to 5% of the population with the greatest increase being in obese people who increased from 2.9% to 10%. Now, with the newer and tougher standards of definition, I am sure that it is much greater than 10%.

"Diabetes" and "prediabetes" are defined below:

At present the diagnosis of Diabetes Mellitus is made by having two fasting blood sugars 126 or above.

The word "mellitus" means "sweet tasting." Thank goodness they have discovered better ways of testing urine for glucose because the doctor used to have to taste the urine to make the diagnosis.

What do you mean "good old days"?

My office assistants, Betty, Debbie and Sheila, are aware that that would be their job if we were still taste-testing. They are VERY happy to have the newer technology in place.

"Prediabetes" is diagnosed by having two fasting blood sugars of 100 or above but less than 126.

When the numbers for the blood sugar values needed for these diagnoses were decreased, the number of diagnosed diabetics increased tremendously.

Why were the numbers changed?

Why will the numbers continue to be changed?

These changes are made every once in a while when it has been found that the complications of diabetes are happening at lower blood glucose levels than what were previously included in the diabetic range. I will discuss the complications of diabetes later.

You will be hearing a term called hemoglobin A-1c. This is an important measurement and will be abbreviated HbA1c. We can tell from moment to moment exactly how our blood sugars are doing just by doing our simple blood checks. But what about while we are sleeping or are at work when we are not likely to check? There is a way to average all of these numbers out and give us a number showing how good or how bad our control has been over the past 30 days. This is done by measuring a chemical substance that has been hooked on to the red blood cells during that 30-day period of time. If the sugars have been high most of the time, this test will be high too. It is a fact that lots of diabetics who claim to have their blood sugars looking "really great" end up with a not-so-great HbA1c. That would mean that some changes need to be made in their diabetes management. It is felt that good control in diabetes is happening when the HbA1c is seven or less. So, if a person has a HbA1c of eight, no matter what his/her other blood sugars have been, we know that his/her diabetes is not well controlled and their body will suffer damage from that.

It is estimated that only one out of five diabetics have the HbA1c in the normal range!

That MUST change!

The complications of diabetes that I mentioned above are myriad. All of the problems with the arteries of the heart that we have been discussing are speeded up. Because the arterial system is body-wide, all of the body is really affected in a similar fashion.

You probably are familiar with the very serious problems that the eyes get into with a condition called "diabetic retinopathy." In this disease the fine little arterioles in the back of the eye (retina) start growing wildly and develop little hemorrhages and microaneurysms (bulges in the artery). This process starts to destroy the area of cells that the eye uses to register light. This results in a loss of sight. It was reported at the annual meeting of the American Diabetes Association in 2005 that these changes in the retina of the eye were actually being found in people that were in the group that we have labeled "prediabetic." If this turns out to be true, then the definition of diabetes will have to be readjusted, with the cutoff being even lower than it is now. Actually, it is such a problem that for every 1% increase in the HbA1c the retinopathy almost doubles!

Similarly the kidneys are damaged by diabetes so that they can no longer expel the waste products of the body. Things can get so bad that the patients sometimes have to have dialysis where a machine (dialysis) actually extracts waste products from the blood and thus preserves life. Diabetes turns out to be the most common single reason for end-stage (end of the line) kidney disease. Because there are so many Type 2 diabetics compared to Type 1's, one-half of all end-stage renal disease will be comprised of Type 2 diabetics. It is estimated that 20-40 percent of all Type 2 diabetics will go on to end-stage renal disease. This is really serious stuff, and anyone who is even at risk of BECOMING a diabetic really ought to give some serious thought about the possible consequences before ever again entering a fast-food joint.

This problem of renal failure in diabetics is so important that more needs to be said about it. It has been found that by improving the blood pressure in a diabetic many of the complications will decrease. In fact, for every 10 mm decrease in blood pressure, there was a 12% decrease in complications of diabetes including renal failure. For example, dropping a blood pressure from 132/80 to 120/72 would cut the diabetic's complications by 12%. That is definitely a lifesaver!

The feet and legs are also affected in many diabetics. The nerves that go to the feet may be damaged by diabetes so that the feet lose the senses of touch and pain. This is labeled "diabetic neuropathy." This is a serious problem and not at all unusual. In fact, for a lot of my diabetics, it becomes the first complication of the disease to rear its ugly head. A diabetic can be walking around for days with a tack in his/her foot and not know it. The first indication of a problem might be the swelling and red streak from the resulting infection.

The arteries of the legs might also be affected, just like those in the heart. They follow the same rules with the endothelium being the key to guarding their welfare. When they become blocked, the legs can experience pain with exercise just like angina of the heart. So, if a person walked a block and experienced pain in the calf of the leg, with the pain subsiding when he/she sat down and rested, that pain would qualify as possibly being caused by one or more artery blockages and would call for further testing.

This condition is termed "peripheral artery disease." New procedures are being developed all the time on how to correct it, but just like the heart, PREVENTION is still the best way to go.

Certainly, if the leg pain were the first symptom one had and it proved to be due to arteriosclerosis, it would call for a checkup of the heart and kidneys. The arterial system consists of one big line. What affects one part will surely affect all of them.

There was a study that compared blood sugar versus blood pressure control. It was found that complications were more reduced by keeping the blood pressure well controlled than by the blood sugar control.

So you see how important it is for diabetics to follow very closely with their doctors to try to prevent these dastardly "complications."

If all of the problems listed above aren't enough, at the 70th annual meeting of the American College of Gastroenterology, a study that took place over a seven-year period of time was presented that involved almost 227,000 subjects. This study did show that having diabetes definitely does increase one's risk of developing colon cancer. At the present time it is suggested that colonoscopy screening start at age 50. Certainly, if there is any family history of colon cancer, I would suggest starting earlier. We should continue to monitor the recommendations as to when to start the colonoscopies.

There is a class of drugs called the ACE Inhibitors. Examples of this group include: Accupril, Capoten, Monopril, and Zestril. The ACEs are known to reduce the amount of protein in the urine of diabetics as the kidneys begin to get into trouble from diabetes, and probably also from hypertension. It was not known for a long time whether this improved the long-term outlook for these diabetics or not.

A study has now been done which shows that kidney complications can be slowed down by the use of one of the ACE Inhibitors. As a result, all diabetics who have kidney tests (Protein in the urine, BUN, and Creatinine, among others) that show that the kidneys are getting into trouble should probably be taking one of these drugs. Unfortunately, there are some possible side effects; one of which is a cough, of all things. Many people have to discontinue the drug because of that. Fortunately, the Angiotensin II Receptor Antagonists mentioned below do not have a cough as a side effect and do have a similar profile of kidney protection.

The Angiotensin II Receptor Antagonists include: Cozaar and Hyzaar. They get about the same results as the ACE Inhibitors but differ in their mode of action. The researchers are at this time looking at these drugs to see if there is an advantage to using the two drugs together. That has not clearly been decided.

Types of Diabetes

There are two types of diabetes. The first is Type 1 Diabetes Mellitus. These are people that are insulin dependent. That means, at the present time, that they are not helped by the various oral medications that are on the market. If they were to use the pills, they would gradually waste away and die. So, for them, injectable insulin is essential for life. There are several different types of insulin on the market now so that good control, that is that the blood glucose levels in the blood do not get too high or too low, is generally possible. Some of the types of insulin are long lasting so that one injection may last in the body for a full 24 hours. This would give smooth control except right after meals at which time the glucose levels jump up. To smooth this out there are "pens" and other injectables some of which are preloaded with very short-acting insulins. These are injected after every good-sized meal. As a result the glucose numbers level out.

Why the big fuss about normal glucose levels?

It is known that the damage that happens from high blood sugars happens 20-30 minutes after eating. We want those values kept as low as we safely can. Go too low and the patient will suffer from hypoglycemia.

The body has a great way of maintaining normal glucose levels. When you eat a meal, the brain senses the increase in blood sugar and immediately the pancreas is ordered to release insulin and presto! The blood sugar (glucose level) comes down. Now, if the pancreas has been damaged by a viral infection or some other similar infection, the pancreas may not respond by producing insulin and you have a Type 1 diabetic.

But, let's say that the pancreas responds just fine. It kicks just the right amount of insulin into the blood stream. But, what if, Heaven forbid, the body cannot use the insulin and the blood sugar remains elevated?

Then you have a Type 2 diabetic. Ninety (90) percent of all diabetics are Type 2.

Well, you say, why can't the body utilize insulin?

Most of the people in this category are overweight. There's that nasty word again! The fat cells get in the way of proper glucose use. Fat does increase the body's resistance to insulin, so it makes sense that this process is called "insulin resistance." So the body puts out more insulin to try to bring down and control blood sugars. This increased insulin level has many side effects...all of them bad. Unfortunately, one of them is weight gain. When it cannot increase any further, the blood sugar elevates and we have the conditions of diabetes or prediabetes as described above. These people can really improve their diabetes management by losing weight, and it is very gratifying when they do. But if their sugars are very high, they may have to be started on the oral medications that are available. These medicines are of several different types and have several modes of action that help the body to utilize its own insulin. Or, the medication may push the pancreas to produce more insulin than it currently is producing.

You cannot take insulin by mouth. The stomach acids destroy it. But our researchers are working on that one, and maybe someday that might become possible. At this time an insulin nasal spray has been approved that should work on both types of diabetes. This is a short-acting preparation that is, at present, used three times a day with meals to take care of the rises in blood sugar that happen when the person eats. It is too early to tell where that will fit into the total treatment program. So, at the present time, many Type 2 diabetics can be controlled on the pills and diet alone.

Unfortunately, with aging, the medicines do not work quite so well and more medications need to be added to keep the blood sugar within desirable limits. As time goes on, they may need to go onto insulin injections.

For many of my Type 2 patients, insulin has turned out to be a good thing. They have found that there is great satisfaction in having good diabetic control without taking all of those pills every day. The insulins nowadays are "human" which means that they are genetically engineered from human cells so that there is no longer any chance of a reaction. That wasn't always the case. Early insulins were pork-based. Sometimes the body didn't like that too well and the patient had reactions. Those shots were also painful because there were some impurities still left in the insulin material.

It has been said that insulin is the most effective but most underused therapy for Type 2 diabetes. Starting it earlier might decrease the risk of many complications.

Under what conditions might you end up on insulin?

Let's take an example. Let's say that you are a Type 2 diabetic. The doctor, after looking into your eye grounds (the back of your eye), states that there are early signs of diabetic retinopathy.

Your urine, when checked, shows that you have 1+ protein (not a lot but any protein is too much protein).

You are on maximum doses of three medications. You have been doing pretty well on your diet. Your HbA1c is 8.6.

Looking at this bunch of results, we see that there probably are kidney changes present from the diabetes. Your eye-grounds show that the diabetes is affecting the vessels in your eyes. There is one thing that you can bank on. If the blood vessels in one part of the body are showing changes, the blood vessels in the whole body are being affected. Your HbA1c is not good, meaning that your diabetes is not under good control.

If at that point your doctor hasn't insisted that you switch over to insulin, then you should strongly suggest that you would like to make that switch. Your future depends on it. Blindness and kidney failure are two very obvious threats to you. You cannot afford to fiddle with oral medications any longer.

I would like to reinforce once again that a normal HbA1c is not above seven.

The interest in and definition of Prediabetes has only happened relatively recently. In a study called the Diabetes Prevention Program, over 3,000 individuals were followed. It was found that 30 minutes of exercise per day, five days a week, along with a healthy diet (low fat, low calorie), reduced the risk of the prediabetics becoming diabetic by 58%. In the same study some of the oral diabetes medications were used on the prediabetics, and these did show a lessening of the number of people going on to frank diabetes. But at present not enough is known about this to justify their use until more studies look at possible problems associated with them. So, for now, the prediabetic's best bet is to hit the diet and exercise, lose some excess weight, and watch the blood sugar levels closely.

The risk of becoming a diabetic increases with each year of getting older, so that in the group 60 and older 18 % of the population has become diabetic. Two things are at work here to cause this. This nasty insulin resistance is present mostly because of the overweight. Also, with aging, the pancreas cuts down on insulin production just like so many other organs in the body decrease their production as the body ages. These two things combine to give you elevated blood sugars.

It is important to note, again, that the damage that happens to the body happens within 30 minutes of eating a meal. The blood sugar goes scooting up as soon as you eat. This is where the "glycemic index" (GI) comes in. The proponents of GI being part of an important strategy in both healthful eating and in diabetes management recognize that the blood sugar is going to rise at different speeds depending on how rapidly the sugars get into the circulation.

For example, you can imagine how quickly the sugars from a candy bar or a bottle of pop would get into the blood stream and cause an elevation of the blood sugar compared with the same number of calories gotten from whole grain bread or oatmeal cookies. We will discuss "glycemic index" later.

Of late it has been found that the distinction between the types of diabetes are blurring. Some of the Type 1 diabetics have gained enough weight that they are insulin resistant, which generally defines Type 2 diabetes. It has also been found that Type 2 diabetics have sometimes gone into diabetic ketoacidosis, a finding that is generally a hallmark of Type 1 diabetes. Studies continue on how to classify these patients. It has been found that when a Type 2 diabetic starts medication he not only has insulin resistance, but he has also lost one-half of the beta cells that produce insulin in the pancreas.

Metabolic Syndrome

You will hear the term Metabolic Syndrome more and more in the coming years. Why? We are now the world's fattest nation! It is as simple as that. The statistics on this condition are staggering. At age 20 in the US, 7% of the population already have the Metabolic Syndrome, and 40% will have it by the age of 60. Eighty (80) percent of the people with diabetes will have it. And, the statistics are worsening each year.

The group of conditions that make up this syndrome include: central obesity, insulin resistance, glucose intolerance, hypertension and dyslipidemia (elevated fats in the blood). The conditions that make up this syndrome may differ a bit according to whose report you are reading. There is still a lot of controversy among physicians about just how important it is to name the syndrome in the first place. The American Heart Association published their revisions in their journal of 9/13/2005. They stated that to make the diagnosis the syndrome must include:

…Elevated waist circumference (abdominal obesity)

…Elevated triglycerides

…Reduced HDL

…Elevated blood pressure

…Elevated fasting blood sugar

Any individual that has three or more of the above has the syndrome by definition.

They are all so very important that none of them can be taken lightly.

The problems of heart disease, and other problems, are worse when this particular group of things are all present at one time in one person. We who see these people in the office know that when a patient has any two of them the probability of potential complications really increases.

We will take a look at each of these conditions.

Central Obesity

…That means that the fat is around your middle. This is an indication that the mesentery holding your intestines in place is loaded with fat along with the obvious fat layer below the skin. The liver also gets a fatty infiltration that reduces its ability to do its job. This has been found to bode worse for the patient than if the fat was around the hip region.

The upper limits of "normal" above, which one qualifies as having central obesity, is 40 inches in men and 35 inches for women.

The triglycerides are fats in the blood. This is one of the things that we test for on the lipid panel. The AHA says that this number should be less than 150. For more on that see Chapter 7, which covers laboratory testing.

The HDL is the "good" stuff and is also a part of the lipid panel that we do routinely. Limits of 40 for men and 50 for women have been set. Anyone below those numbers qualifies in the definition of the syndrome.

Blood pressure standards are a little over-generous I think. They are set at or above 130/85 as the values to qualify in the syndrome. That low number (diastolic) of 85 is much higher than where I want YOU to be.

The blood sugar cutoff was set at or above 100 on a fasting glucose. We know that an FBS of 100 qualifies a person for a diagnosis of "prediabetes" now.

Insulin Resistance

This business of insulin resistance is gaining importance because it is the problem behind most Type 2 diabetics. It means that the body, for one reason or another, cannot use the insulin that is present. As mentioned previously, the most frequent reason for this is obesity.

Hypertension

You certainly know what that is…or do you? I say it that way because the definition changes fairly frequently as investigators find out more about the complications of high blood pressure, and at what level of blood pressure these complications are likely to occur. The present definition is a blood pressure that is above 130/85.

Glucose Intolerance

This is a term that you will hear more frequently also. This simply means that your body is not handling the sugars, as it should. For example, the pregnant female may have a "modified glucose tolerance test." Her fasting blood sugar on a single sample may be normal. She is then given a measured amount of glucose by mouth. Her blood will be checked a few hours later to see if her body was able to respond to the glucose with insulin production from the pancreas enough to bring the blood sugar down into the range that it is supposed to be. If her blood sugar has not returned to normal two hours after drinking the glucose, by definition she would have "impaired glucose tolerance" and will be treated until the end of the pregnancy. This will have value in being sure that the pregnancy goes to completion without complication.

Medications that are used in diabetes

All of the drugs mentioned in this book are mentioned in "overview" form. This is not meant to tell you how or if to take the medications. So, of course, the patient would need to discuss dosages, drug interactions, complications and side effects, etc., with their doctor before taking any of them.

We have discussed insulin resistance. The nicest way of attacking that would be to lose weight, shape up, and be a healthier person. Then, hopefully, you could sit back and watch the blood tests all improve. For those that are not able to do that, there are some medications that actually lessen the insulin resistance. Some of the medications actually work on the liver to cut down on its production of sugar. More and more doctors are finding it necessary to use more than one type of medication at a time in order to get the very best glucose control that is possible. The rewards are certainly there for bringing the blood sugars down to as near to normal as possible.

Remember that you can't take insulin by mouth because it would be destroyed in the stomach. Thus our oral blood sugar control has to be brought about by fiddling with the liver and various other organs.

The first group of oral medications that was available for diabetes was the sulfonourea class.

The sulfonourea class includes Diabeta, Diabinese, and Glucotrol along with other medications. This group of medicines pushes the pancreas to produce a bit more insulin. That may work up to a certain point. There comes a time when this medication just doesn't work anymore. This is because the pancreas has been pushed to its limit. Raising the dosage usually will not help a lot at that point.

The main side effect has been hypoglycemia (low blood sugar). So the doctor usually starts out with a low dosage and works the dose up as needed.

Allergy-wise this is a sulfa product so that one would not use it if he/she were allergic to sulfa. These drugs have been used for over forty years and they still work AND they are cheap.

Then there is the biguanide class of medicine. The only representative of this class at the present time is Metformin. It works mostly by decreasing the production of glucose by the liver. It has been around since the 1990s.

It should not be used in people with decreased renal (kidney) function. Big problems (lactic acidosis) can result in those people. But other than that it turns out to be pretty safe and is well tolerated for most everyone who needs it. Many of the treatments for diabetes tend to make a patient gain weight. Most of the diabetics certainly do not need that. Metformin has the tendency to allow the patient to maintain their weight or maybe even lose some.

The major side effect other than lactic acidosis is related to gastrointestinal upset. Lower dosing at the start will sometimes prevent the GI side effects from happening. Then one can often successfully increase the dose without a problem.

Another group of medications is the thiazolidinediones (TZDs). Avandia and Actos are representatives of this class of drugs.

The TZDs work by increasing the body's ability to utilize the insulin that is already there. This may be especially helpful in the overweight diabetic since it works mostly in areas other than the liver. These other areas, fat and muscle, are the areas that make the overweight patients so insulin resistant (insulin just doesn't work properly). This pill partially overcomes that resistance. This allows those tissues to use the insulin. Thus the level of glucose circulating in the blood is lowered. This, as we have seen, cuts down on the body's tendency to load up fat cells when there is an excess of sugar floating around in the bloodstream.

In 2005 the American Heart Association announced that a study using Actos showed that it reduced the risk of a second heart attack by 28% in people who had already had a heart attack.

One side effect of the TZDs, especially when it is used along with insulin, is the formation of edema (swelling). For that reason it would be used only with great care in people who have heart failure where edema can become life threatening. Because the liver sometimes is injured by the TZDs, it is important to run liver blood tests during the first year of taking this medication.

Another group of diabetic medications is the meglitinides. An example of this class is Starlix.

This group stimulates the pancreas to produce insulin a lot like the sulfonoureas. These have a short span of action, so they are generally used along with some longer-acting drug such as Metformin. They are taken three times a day before meals, and they are intended to reduce that spike of blood sugar that happens when we eat a meal.

Alpha-glucosidase inhibitors are represented by Glyset.

This drug is given with each meal in order to reduce the upward swings of glucose when you eat. It usually would be used in conjunction with a longer-acting medication such as a sulfonourea. Remember that the upward swing when you eat is what causes a lot of the problems in diabetes.

The newest of the diabetes drugs is in a class called the incretin mimetics.

The lone representative at this time is Byetta. This drug is given by injection twice a day. A pill form of this drug is in the works for the future. Interestingly, it will bring blood sugar down if the blood sugar is elevated and will not change the blood sugar if it is not elevated. What a neat drug family this promises to be! Impressive weight losses are reported.

Studies have shown a delay on the treating doctor's part. Some doctors are just too slow in making adjustments to the medications of diabetics. Studies have shown that there are diabetics with HbA1c of 8.4, for instance, and when checked by investigators a year later, they are still on the same medications and the HbA1c hasn't changed!

If the HbA1c is not in the 7's or below, the diabetes is NOT in good control. If your HbA1c is not 7 or below, you should be seen every three months and your medications should be changed, or some change in what you are doing should be accomplished. Why? It is because the body is being damaged during this time. We cannot stop the ticking clock of cellular damage that happen, but we can slow it down.

Chapter 6—Obesity; Inflammation

I want to have a good body, but not as much as I want dessert.

Jason Love

The US is the fattest nation in the world!

The amount of fat that we carry around with us really impacts on our lives. As you look at the various chapters in this book, you will see obesity mentioned in almost every one.

The risk of diabetes increases dramatically with weight gain. As weight is gained, the arteries become stiffer and the blood pressure goes up. When the blood pressure goes up, the risk of stroke, heart attack and kidney damage start to increase, so there are lots of good reasons not to be overweight.

Abdominal obesity carries some especially bad outcomes with it. There is obviously fat in the abdomen, but there is also fat in the liver in this condition. This fat reduces the liver's ability to remove insulin. Insulin has been known to constrict arteries. This leads towards troubles with the heart.

There are some suggestions for weight loss in this book. They are scattered around but are mostly in the "Diet" chapter.

Years ago, when I wished to lose a few pounds, it really was fairly easy to do. I simply went on a low calorie diet with three small meals a day instead of three large ones. In about one week or less, I no longer was hungry after a small meal. I figured that the stomach had actually shrunk down in size so that it would not hold as much before feeling "full."

That balloon was shot down when I saw X-ray studies that showed that the stomach did not actually shrink down in that period of time.

OK. Well, anyway, it worked for me.

There is an interesting phenomenon going on now along that line in our society.

People who are morbidly obese and are otherwise in good shape can have their stomach "stapled" or have a "gastric bypass." A BMI of 40 or above is generally required, except in special circumstances.

In the stomach stapling procedure, staples are placed in the stomach, usually using a 'scope. Only a small pocket is left to act as a stomach for food. These folks REALLY get a full feeling fast. In this procedure the stomach has just been made smaller with no other changes. When these folks get home, they are placed on exactly measured amounts of food so as not to stretch the stomach out again. If they do stretch it out again, all of the previous benefit is lost and they resume their weight gain. Interestingly, the surgeons do not allow much water during meals because of the risk of stretching the stomach out again. If they do not stretch it out again, the weight loss is fantastic and they become "new" people as the pounds melt away.

A "success" is when the patient loses 50% of their excess weight and keeps it off for five years. With this procedure, 80% achieve some weight loss and 30% achieve a normal weight. Half of the patients will have regained their lost weight after five years.

Some have the procedure done again.

In the gastric bypass procedure the stomach is made smaller, and the first portion of the small bowel is bypassed. This cuts down on the amount of bowel that can pick up nutrients and calories. Because of the problems of possible malnutrition and vitamin deficiency that come as a result, this procedure is more fraught with problems.

These procedures have lots of risks associated with them, and they are last-resort procedures when all else has failed and the patient's life depends on them. There is a mortality rate associated with both procedures of around 1.5%. As usual, this rate varies, usually depending on the number of these procedures the surgeon has done in the past, along with the health status of the patient. The more experienced the surgeon, the better the outcome. So, if you plan to have this procedure done, be sure that there is no alternative. Also, make sure that you get the most experienced surgeon possible. (Medical Center?)

If you happen to be overweight, you might try the frequent SMALL meals and see if it works for YOU without the surgery.

An interesting finding is being reported which may explain why so many things go sour when a person is obese. Studies were done that suggest that being obese accelerates aging. If this turns out to be true, it would explain so many things. The report is being criticized and talked about. It will set off a lot of experimentation.

You may be interested in how the researchers arrived at this conclusion.

It seems that when one looks at chromosomes there are little particles out on the end of the chromosomes called "telomeres." We begin life with long telomeres, and this part shortens with age and damage. The length of the telomere thus provides an age estimate of the cell that it came from.

When the researchers looked at the lifestyles of the cells' owners, they found a huge difference in cell age. An obese person's cells were 8.8 years older than the lean person. A smoker was 4.6 years older than a non-smoker. If you take an obese smoker who has smoked 20 cigarettes a day for 40 years, the age difference is 10 years!

It is noted that the chromosomes that they looked at were from white blood cells. It remains to be seen if these findings hold true for the rest of the body's cells. The investigator notes that when the telomeres get too short to divide any more the game is over. The clock has run out. From his studies, the telomeres in men seem to "run out" about 7 years before they do in women. It is known that women, on the average, live 7.4 years longer than men. So, at this time, this method of investigation seems to hold some promise.

The author feels that damage to the telomeres is probably caused by "oxidative free radicals." These are discussed elsewhere in the book. Smoking and obesity are known to produce oxidative free radicals.

The effects seem to be permanent. Stopping smoking and losing weight may reduce the effects but cannot restore them.

How do you know where you stand on the obesity scale?

One way is to find your Body Mass Index (BMI). To calculate it yourself you simply take your height in inches times itself. Divide this number into your weight in pounds, and then multiply the result by 703.

The Center for Disease Control uses the following BMI definitions:

Below 18.5	underweight
$18.5 \rightarrow 24.9$	normal
$25 \rightarrow 29.9$	overweight
30 and above	obese

When a person's BMI is above normal, the CDC states that their risk of having the following conditions increases:

Premature death

Cardiovascular disease

High blood pressure

Osteoarthritis

Some cancers

Diabetes Mellitus

It should be noted that on certain individuals this rule does not hold true. The very muscular person may have a high weight but a perfectly normal abdominal measurement. He or she should be considered normal.

Getting weight off and keeping weight off are real challenges, but there are people who do it every day. The National Weight Control Registry is a research study of people who have succeeded at long-term weight loss. Its members include thousands of Americans who have lost and kept off at least 30 pounds for more than six years.

They report taking these steps to avoid gaining weight:

…Exercise regularly. Walk four miles a day or burn the equivalent in calories in some other form of exercise.

…Limit calories to 1800 per day.

…Consume a relatively low-fat diet and have breakfast daily.

…Weigh regularly.

…Eat in a consistent way. Don't pig-out on special occasions.

…Keep a record of how much is eaten and of weights.

Makes sense to me.

We have listed a bunch of reasons above for why one would like not to be obese. Let's add another. The National Cancer Institute has begun a major research project to try to determine why it is that obese people have a higher cancer rate than the non-obese. The NCI will be providing funding of $54 million to four centers to carry out a five-year investigation. Hopefully, this will get the public's attention as to the importance of not being overweight. Keep tuned in.

Chapter 7—The Laboratory Tests and What They Mean

If one could give every individual the right amount of nourishment and exercise, not too little and not too much, we would have found the safest way to health.

Hippocrates

For this, most of you will need to visit your favorite doctor and have some blood drawn. This may have already been done and if so congratulations! If not, it's time to get it done.

Fasting Blood Sugar (FBS)

Because so many problems come as a result of being overweight and of being diabetic, I have placed this test as number one. I think that you MUST know your blood glucose level. The more overweight that you are, the more urgent it is that the test be done. If you have a family history of diabetes, it also increases the urgency of getting it done. At the present time, values of 126 or above are diagnostic of "Diabetes Mellitus." Values from 100 to 125 are diagnostic of "Prediabetes."

So what does one do if he/she has a value of 98?

What would you do?

That number is trouble. The first two places to look are:

1) Am I overweight? Just dropping five pounds will make a huge difference.

2) How is my diet?

If one is taking in a lot of carbohydrates with snacks, fast foods, etc., just making a diet change will improve the testing.

For more info, see the section on Diabetes, found in Chapter 5.

Hemoglobin A1c

Diabetics will need to be followed with this test. It currently is not being used in making the diagnosis of diabetes. What it does is average out the blood sugar concentrations over the past 30 days prior to the blood being drawn. The blood glucose levels in the two weeks prior to the blood drawing weigh most heavily in the result. The reason that HbA1c is so important is that fasting blood sugars only give a value of how your blood glucose level is at any one instant in time. The "average" that the HbA1c gives takes a lot of guesswork out of diabetes care. We all might tend to not remember the undesirable home glucose monitoring numbers that we have gotten and just remember the good ones. For example, many are the times that a patient has told me that their home monitoring values are "just swell, doc" only to find that they have a lousy HbA1c.

That's just human nature.

It has been shown that keeping a HbA1c at seven or below will reduce the incidence of diabetic complications to the eyes, kidneys, nerves and more.

It is important for the patient to get to that magic number seven or below. Medications and lifestyle need to keep being changed and adjusted until that seven is obtained. To do otherwise is asking for all sorts of nasty complications.

The test is done using the red cells in the blood. Scientists have found that a substance in the red cells called "glycosolated hemoglobin" provides a mirror of how the glucose levels have been over the past month.

The Lipid Panel

The guidelines at present state that everyone should have a complete lipid panel by age 20, and the panel should be repeated every five years unless, because of problems, the panel needs to be repeated sooner.

I guess that my personal feeling on this is that age 20 is a bit late. We know that by the late teens many people already have fatty deposits in their arteries. I think that it would make more sense to check the children at least by the time that they enter high school in order to try to find any problem as early as possible. Especially, as we see more of the children becoming overweight, or downright obese, their risks of having correctable problems increase. Also, if the kids have a family history of diabetes, heart disease, or stroke, it would make sense not to wait until after high school to find out if their genes are going to be, or already are, a problem.

The usual basic testing includes HDL, LDL, Total Cholesterol, and Serum Triglycerides.

Low Density Lipoprotein (LDL)

Lipoproteins are combinations of fat and protein produced by your body. Their usefulness is that they can deliver some fats into the bloodstream to your cells, which need the fats. These fats do not dissolve in the blood, and thus would otherwise not be available to be taken up by the cells of the body.

The LDL is the "bad guy." There is a lot of it in the blood stream, and it is the culprit that is behind the blockages and masses of fatty deposits under the surface of our arteries that we talk so much about.

As for what are the "normal" values for LDL, you will find figures that are "risk-stratified." For instance, for a healthy person who is "low risk," the "normal" might be an LDL of up to 130. But, for a person with diabetes and heart disease, the goal may be to get that number way down to 100 or below! The problem here is that darned near all of us are going to have arteriosclerosis during our lifetime, so how much water does the stratification hold? As a result, I feel that this "stratification" has some flaws and that we ALL should have as our goal getting that number down as low as possible (70?).

I am not alone in this thinking. I have already mentioned that there are some doctors that believe that the statins should be sold over the counter so that EVERYONE can take their daily statin along with their vitamin pill every morning. For more on that see a book by Peter Salgo, MD called *The Heart of The Matter*. Dr. Salgo is an experienced Intensive Care doctor who daily witnesses the carnage that results from what is so nonchalantly labeled "heart disease." The term doesn't even come close to describing the human suffering and misery that is associated with it.

I disagree on statins over-the-counter at this time, but agree that the goals in therapy are lagging behind where they really need to be. I am sure the "powers that be" will gradually change their recommendations to get these numbers lower and lower until they finally come to the conclusion that I have just stated. No one should be satisfied with an LDL of 130 at this time. I believe that the problem has been that these findings concerning LDL are fairly recent, and those higher figures are just way points on the way down to really good numbers.

How low can you go? There are some few lucky people out there that have LDLs in the 60s with no drugs or special measures being used. Great genes! (See "Putting It All Together" chapter.) One observation if I may…I have never found one of these people to be much overweight, so they probably have pretty great health habits along with the genes.

Note: As these numbers that define where your test results should be get pushed lower and lower, it becomes more and more difficult to attain them. One cannot be a couch potato and expect it to happen, no matter what else is being done.

High Density Lipoprotein (HDL)

HDL plays a huge role in keeping us healthy and in keeping those pipes open. There are some very fortunate people out there that have high HDLs, usually women. When they have HDLs of 75 or above (called the Longevity Syndrome), they live five to seven years longer than their-age mates. It is not certain at this point how important the LDL is for these people. Studies have been inconclusive.

We have been discussing a lot about the nasty LDL. Well, HDL can actually remove the nasty stuff, as we discussed earlier. The entire process of how it does that gets a little sticky, and the researchers are still working on it. Basically, HDL has the ability to pick up and transport cholesterol from the tissues and then transport it back to the liver. This is called "Reverse Cholesterol

Transport." In the liver it undergoes some processing. Research is still going on as to where the resulting substances end up.

For people whose HDL is below the standard "normal," the drugs that we have are not really good at correcting it. Exercise is one of the most efficient ways of increasing it and in keeping it up. This is another good reason to have a good exercise program in place.

Total Cholesterol

This started out years ago as being the test that we really concentrated on. It was the only test that we had in the lipid family. We knew that when this was high the person had a health problem that might well lead to his/her death or disability.

Now, however, we have all sorts of other testing that we can do to more specifically pinpoint the problems in our vessels. The total cholesterol test is included in the panel of tests that we order. But anymore, it is just a test that sort of "goes along with" the others in determining how much or how little of a problem there is.

At the time of this writing, the official recommendation is that this number be below 200. The number 170 is being considered as more desirable. You should certainly use 170 or below as the values that you shoot for because anything 200 or above certainly is trouble.

When a number such as this is elevated, it is important that once action is taken that repeat testing is done every three to four months to be sure that things are improving. As mentioned previously, LDL is now the part of the lipid panel that is most used for normalization or for correction of the lipid panel.

Triglycerides

Triglycerides are the chemical forms in which most fats exist in food as well as in the body. They are also present in blood plasma and, in association with cholesterol, form the "plasma lipids."

Triglycerides in plasma are derived from fats eaten in foods or made in the body from other energy sources such as carbohydrates.

Calories ingested in a meal that are not used immediately by tissues are converted to triglycerides and transported to fat cells to be stored. Hormones regulate the release of triglycerides from fat tissues so that they meet the body's needs for energy between meals. When one has an excess of triglycerides in the blood plasma, it is labeled "hypertriglyceridemia." This is linked to the occurrence of coronary artery disease in some people. Elevated triglycerides may be a consequence of other diseases such as untreated Diabetes Mellitus.

At present, the "normal" values are as follows. These measurements are made after an overnight fast:

Normal	Less than 150 mgm/dl
Borderline-high	150 to 199 mgm/dl
High	200 to 499 mgm/dl
Very high	500 mgm/dl or above

Occasionally you find a person who has REALLY elevated triglycerides. Usually they do not have any symptoms. The condition is usually found on a routine blood test. They can have Triglycerides of over 1000! This is a very serious matter. When working as a laboratory technician in the past, I often was able to make the diagnosis of "hypertriglyceridemia" by just looking at the blood. When you look at their serum (blood without the blood clot), it looks like milk because it is so loaded with these fat globules. (By the way that's the way your serum appears after eating a fatty meal.) You can imagine how your body feels about that! The serum from a person who hasn't eaten in 12 hours should be sparkling clear and yellow.

The people who have very high triglycerides usually have a genetic problem that predisposes them to this, and their family members certainly should get tested.

As you can imagine, the risk of atherosclerosis with all its problems is certainly elevated in these people.

But there is a more urgent problem when the triglycerides are this elevated. The pancreas can get inflamed and this results in "pancreatitis." This is a problem you would not wish on your worst enemy. Well…maybe you would.

Anyway, when the pancreas gets inflamed, it causes a SEVERE abdominal pain. There is no quick cure. The patient is placed on IV fluids for hydration and is given pain medications until the pain subsides. Then we use medications that reduce the level of triglycerides in the blood. Some of these patients go on to develop a "chronic pancreatitis" and, like it sounds, this consists of recurrent bouts of this severe pain.

So it is difficult to imagine a better reason to know your triglyceride level.

The following are the American Heart Association Dietary Treatment Goals for Hypertriglyceridemia:

"Changes in lifestyle are the main therapy for hypertriglyceridemia. These are:

…If you are overweight, cut down on calories to reach your ideal body weight. This includes all sources of calories, from fats, proteins, carbohydrates and alcohol.

…Reduce the saturated fat and cholesterol content of your diet.

…Reduce the intake of alcohol considerably. Even small amounts of alcohol can lead to large changes in triglyceride levels.

…Be physically active for at least thirty minutes on most or all days each week.

…People with high triglycerides may need to substitute monounsaturated and polyunsaturated fats—such as those found in canola oil, olive oil or liquid margarine—for saturated fats. Substituting carbohydrates for fats may raise triglyceride levels and may decrease HDL (good) cholesterol in some people.

…Substitute fish high in Omega-3 fatty acids instead of meats high in saturated fats like hamburger. Fatty fish like mackerel, lake trout, herring, sardines, albacore tuna, and salmon are high in Omega-3 fatty acids.

Because other risk factors for coronary artery disease multiply the hazard from hypertriglyceridemia, control high blood pressure and avoid cigarette smoking. If drugs are used to treat hypertriglyceridemia, dietary management is still important. Patients should follow the specific plans laid out by their physicians and nutritionists."

Ratio Total/HDL Cholesterol

When you obtain your Lipid Panel, you may see this ratio as part of the report. If it is not there, it is really easy to calculate so don't hesitate to do it on your own. It is a simple division. You take the total cholesterol number and divide it by the HDL level.

There, that was easy.

If the resulting number is three point something or less, it can be considered normal. If it is four or above, in my opinion, it is NOT normal and you need to figure out how to change it.

Example: If a person has Total Cholesterol of 200 and HDL of 35, when we make the division, we get a ratio of 5.7. We knew it would not be good because of the low HDL level and the not-so-good Total Cholesterol level. This person must try to raise the HDL and lower the Total Cholesterol.

A study was done on women to see if the simple tests like this were as predictive of problems as were the more expensive tests such as C-Reactive Protein and Homocysteine. It was found that the standard tests of Total Cholesterol, HDL, Triglycerides, LDL, and this Ratio were as predictive of trouble as was such tests as the CRP.

C-Reactive Protein

This is a test that, at this time, is not a standard part of the lipid panel. It is being cited in the literature more and more and may soon become a more important part because it is a measure of inflammation. It does not tell you where the inflammation is, but it just points out that it is there.

Certainly, as the role of inflammation in heart disease has long been known, it seems certain that this test will continue to increase in importance. Hopefully, some other test will be developed that will indicate more exactly that the heart is the site of the inflammation. This has happened with a number of other laboratory tests. It just takes a little time for the science boys to scratch their collective heads and come up with better tests for us.

Homocysteine

This test is not widely accepted at the present time as part of the screening that we recommend is done regularly. As more studies come along, that may change. Elevated levels of homocysteine appear to be an independent risk factor for cerebrovascular disease (strokes), peripheral vascular disease (legs), coronary heart disease, and venous thromboembolic disease (clots in veins). So far, it is thought that having high values of this substance doesn't weigh in as heavily as smoking, high blood pressure, or diabetes.

It is known that if you are low on Vitamin B-6, B-12, or Folic Acid that the homocysteine levels will be elevated. The question that remains is whether or not the elevation of the homocysteine CAUSES vessel changes or is just there along with other things that are causing it.

Mass screening has been considered, but no one is exactly sure what to do about the abnormal values when they are found. And if people are treated, no one is exactly sure that the treatment is necessary.

Dr. Liem, in the Netherlands, completed a study on whether low doses of Folic Acid might reduce the Homocysteine level and thus reduce the risk of heart blockage and heart-related death. His study failed to show any difference in coronary disease or its complications.

Another trial done in the Netherlands, called the NORVIT trial, failed to show any benefit of lowering Homocysteine levels in preventing second heart attacks.

There have been many other studies that show that the vitamin supplementation doesn't seem to help when the vascular disease is already present. The question is, will vitamins work in preventing one from having a heart attack?

So, this test may not be dead in the water as yet, but it certainly is getting close to it.

As a result of all this, it is suggested at the present time by most researchers that everyone take a multiple vitamin that has B-6, B-12, and Folic Acid in it and forego mass screening.

It is known that as the body ages it doesn't pick up the B vitamins from food like it did when it was younger. Therefore, vitamin supplementation becomes more important in the elderly.

I take mine every day. You probably should take yours too.

Small Dense LDL

This is not a standard test as yet, but it is rather interesting. The researchers actually have known for a long time that LDL was a "killer." They went one step further and actually measured the particle size of the LDL molecules. What they found was that the LDL particles ranged in size from larger to smaller. They also found that the smaller the particle the more weight it carried in the prediction of the occurrence of coronary artery disease. In one study they found that it was second only to total cholesterol in its ability to predict coronary artery disease. Some day, as new and better testing procedures come along, it may become a major player in the diagnosis of atherosclerosis.

Chapter 8—Smoking: The Evils Thereof

Nicotine patches are great...stick one over each eye and you can't find your cigarettes.

Author unknown

Smoking has really been a problem all over the world. It has increased the amount of heart disease along with all sorts of other problems. The fact is that smokers are TWICE as likely as non-smokers to have heart attacks. It is estimated that about 30% of all heart disease deaths are due to smoking. Twenty-two percent of Americans continue to smoke!

How young can smoking cigarettes affect the arteries of the heart? "Fatty streaks," usually the earliest sign of atherosclerosis in the blood vessels, have been found in the arteries of aborted fetuses of moms who smoked! It hasn't been proven that the smoking was the cause, but it gives reason to wonder, doesn't it?

A report from the Buenos Aires Cardiological Research Institute in 2005 listed fatty streaking in 15 of 16 babies that died of SIDS. They also found coronary lesions on the arteries of 10 of 12 aborted fetuses of smoking moms. There were two fetuses and three SIDS babies whose arteries showed the lesions where the mothers had stated that they did NOT smoke. These findings are building stronger and stronger cases against anyone ever smoking. Until more is known, please caution pregnant ladies about this possible problem.

What can one cigarette do?

With PET Scanning, a lady's heart was scanned two hours after smoking ONE cigarette.

The scan was abnormal. It showed spasm of the coronary arteries! The scan was repeated after the lady was smoking-free for 24 hours. The scan was normal. Think about this the next time that you breathe someone else's cigarette smoke.

This has been documented in other studies. If you are a current smoker, you have twenty times more risk of coronary artery spasm than if you were a non-smoker.

This spontaneous narrowing of the coronary arteries reduces the blood flow to the heart. This can lead to a heart attack (myocardial infarction). To complicate matters, the various chemicals in the smoke lower the amount of oxygen available in the circulating blood. This reduces the oxygen going to various parts of the body, including the heart, just when the heart needs it most.

Smoking turns out to be one of the most awful things that one can do to one's body. When you start to recount the problems that this can bring about, it gets mind-boggling. It is almost to the point at this time that one can name a disease, and it will have been shown that smoking can either be a partial or total cause, or a reason for it to get worse. I will recount some of the problems that come to mind.

We all are familiar with lung cancer. Most of these cases are found in present or past smokers, and guess who has the fastest-rising incidence of lung cancer?

Women!

In my practice, if you show a male an abnormal chest X-ray, or if I advise him that when I listen to his lungs with a stethoscope that his lungs are showing signs of lung disease, there is a pretty good chance that he will stop smoking. The incidence of successful smoking cessation of these men is around 50% in my practice.

Women, however, are a different story. I have a dismal success rate. My success is probably in the 15% range. It is still worth trying, and with each success comes a great deal of reward for all concerned. But why is it such a task for a female to stop smoking?

It is the fear of weight gain. The cigarettes have many additives that result in decreasing the appetite for foods. Without this crutch, the person becomes a "nibbler" and weight gain results.

Not all the news is bad, however. It has been found that as far as heart disease goes, when you stop smoking, you lose that as a risk factor for heart disease.

I can tell by auscultation if a patient has been smoking for five years or more. The damage to the lungs by that time is very real.

Eighty (80) percent of smokers already have abnormal lung findings at five years. This is because they are developing a lung disease called COPD. This stands for Chronic Obstructive Pulmonary Disease. This happens because there is an almost constant inflammation going on in the lungs of a smoker. (Notice the "smoker's cough.") As we have seen, and will see, the body does not do well with chronic inflammation anywhere. This inflammation in the lungs sets the stage for an infection, which leads to thickening of the walls between the air sacs. This is not good. The oxygen that you breathe into your lungs needs to pass through those walls, and the carbon dioxide that your body needs to get rid of also has to pass through the walls for you to be able to exhale it.

As I listen to the lungs of smokers, the breath sounds that I hear get steadily more difficult to hear as the thickness of those walls increases. Less air passes through the lungs as the lungs become stiffer. Symptom-wise, the smoker may first notice that he/she is a little more short of breath than usual when rushing up a flight of stairs. As the disease progresses, so do the symptoms. So that on a "muggy" day it becomes quite a bit more difficult to breathe. This, of course, can progressively worsen so that finally the lungs can no longer supply the amount of oxygen necessary for life while one is breathing room air. At this point, supplemental oxygen has to be started.

So, I have this healthy-appearing male in front of me who has a ten-year smoking history of one pack per day (ten pack years). I have advised this man that I detect early changes of COPD when I auscultate (listen to) his lungs. He asks what happens if he quits smoking now. I advise him that so far there has been no way found of reversing COPD, but if he were to stop smoking now, it would hopefully prevent the disease from worsening. At the same time I advise him of his risk of heart disease becoming less when he stops. Because of changes in the lung sounds, I generally get a chest X-ray at this point to be sure that there is no lung cancer or other problems besides COPD. If the X-ray fails to show early COPD, that's nice, but unfortunately an X-ray just isn't able to pick up COPD in the early stages. So, if an X-ray DOES show COPD, then the COPD is probably no longer in the early stages.

Then I outline a plan to improve the body's ability to breathe. I think at whatever stage COPD is found that specific exercises are called for to strengthen the muscles that the body uses in taking a breath.   There are also medications that can help the person exercise more without getting short of breath. With the increased exercise, the patient can get his body into an improved degree of fitness, thus helping the heart tremendously. Without the increased exercise, the ability to improve lifestyle really suffers.

Bad things continue to surface. A study was done in Canada that followed women who had never smoked but were exposed to long-term PASSIVE smoke. They found that breast cancer was increased in these women by 27%. Note was made that in the studies that collected the most complete measures of passive smoking the observed breast cancer risk was increased by 90%. Some studies, furthermore, showed that in premenopausal women who DO smoke the risk of breast cancer was elevated 108% compared to non-smokers. The comment was made, "It is clearly time to redouble efforts to reduce non-smokers exposure to secondhand smoke in all environments."

Amen!

Chapter 9—Diet; That Much; Rewards;
Glycemic Index

Life is uncertain. Eat dessert first.

Ernestine Ulmer

Lots of my patients would like for me to furnish them with a diet that would guarantee that all of their problems would be solved. They would lose weight, be happy and healthy, and their cholesterol panels would be "just swell."

So sorry. In my opinion that list does not exist. I will give you some general principles to go by and will discuss some really bad stuff along with some "good things." I will not attempt to cover all of the "good" and "bad" foods but will try to hit some high points that have worked for my patients and which I believe are especially important.

We start with a "given." And that is that the body really likes all the "bad stuff" and doesn't care much for a lot of the "good stuff." So there has to be considerable relearning going on in order to take advantage of all that these foods have to offer. This relearning is not meant to set up habits for a day, a week, or a month. They are habits for the rest of your life!

We need to discuss how the body handles the foods that you eat. This book dwells on the evils of fats, and this is why.

The high blood cholesterol, we know, is bad because of its influence on the bringing about of the atherosclerosis in the arteries along with obesity and all that that entails. The fact is that our livers are responsible for producing about 80% of the cholesterol found in our blood. Only about 20% of the cholesterol in our bloodstream comes from what we eat. So, it seems that our major problem here is to cut down on the amount of cholesterol that the liver produces. Therefore, an occasional egg for breakfast is not going to influence the cholesterol level a lot since there is not a lot of fat involved.

When we eat saturated, hydrogenated, or partially hydrogenated fats (bad stuff), the liver turns them into chemical compounds called "acetone units." If we haven't eaten too much fat, these units will be burned as energy. If, however, we have consumed more fat than the body needs for energy, these units will be converted to cholesterol, which may be absorbed later and turned into fat deposits in our bodies.

Some Good Stuff...Beans

One of the most underrated foods, in my opinion, is beans. It is a good food and has high protein content. This is one food that should help you to make that important leap that you are going to make in getting off of your meat diet.

Historically, beans were grown as a food staple 9,000 years ago by the people of Mexico and Peru. Our own Native Americans were growing beans thousands of years ago. They also grew grains, corn and squash, realizing that the foods complemented each other in a healthful diet.

One major problem that beans have, which we all are familiar with, and all have experienced firsthand, is that beans are great gas producers. There is a product on the market called Beano. This product does solve this problem pretty well when used properly. It is simply an enzyme that aids the body in breaking down the beans so that there is less gas production. So, it should not be thought of as a "medicine" but as a digestive aid. No, I don't have any connection to the company. I just think that it is a great product. There are a lot of recipes out there that will also cut down on gas production when beans are on the menu.

Olives

Olives make up a large part of the Mediterranean Diet. This diet has now been shown to work just as well outside the Mediterranean region. The olive has been called one of the world's healthiest foods. The olive itself is very bitter when it comes off the tree. The green olives are picked before they ripen, and the black olives are picked after they ripen. They then undergo various processes, according to the olive type, to make them marketable.

They are a source of iron, vitamin E, and copper. They are 12% dietary fiber. They also provide some good nutrients including oleic, linoleic, and linilenic fatty acids. These are unsaturated fatty acids that the body needs.

Artificial Sweeteners

There are still people out there who haven't made the switch to artificial sweeteners and are adding sugars to their foods. Some have a fear that the sweeteners aren't safe. Others just like the taste of the "real stuff." According to the FDA, the average American eats TWENTY teaspoons of sugar per day! To obtain this number, they included Valentine's Day, year-end holidays, Halloween, and other "excuse" days at which times we tend to eat an excessive amount of the sweets. Nearly 60% of this amount is from sodas and other sweetened drinks. With that awful figure in mind, you know exactly where to look in order to reduce YOUR calorie intake.

If you haven't made the switch over to diet sodas, it is time that you do.

The FDA has now approved five sugar substitutes, including Saccharin (Sweetn' Low), Aspartane (Equal), Acesulfame K (Sweet One, Sunett), Sucralose (Splenda), and Neotame (Nutrasweet).

Fish Oil (Omega 3)

These are polyunsaturated fatty acids. The body is not able to manufacture them, which may make that Omega-3 capsule a bit more valuable.

The original interest in fish oil came about because of the Eskimos. They consume lots of fish of the type that are rich in Omega-3 fatty acids. They also have a low incidence of coronary artery disease. That has been the reason for investigation of the fish oils over the decades.

There has been considerable evidence to support fish oil as a heart disease prevention medication. The stuff has been so difficult to take because of taste and side effects that its popularity has been sort of up and down. As newer methods of production have cut down on the taste problems, fish oil is becoming increasingly used for cardiovascular protection in a capsule form.

There are a number of trials that show beneficial results in Omega 3's effect on heart disease.

One of the trials was the DART (Diet And Reinfarction Trial). This trial was made up of people who had already suffered a myocardial infarction, so we know that these people already had coronary artery disease. One-half of the people were given Omega 3, and the other half of the people did not take the Omega 3. The Omega-3 group later was found to have a 62% reduction in cardiovascular disease death and a 56% reduction in deaths from all causes.

It is still not known for sure how these good benefits happen. There are many theories including the possibility 1) That they cut down on rhythm problems when the heart is injured, 2) That they stimulate endothelial cell-derived nitric oxide, 3) That they decrease platelet aggregation (stickiness), or 4) That they somehow cut down on inflammation.

Oatmeal

The USDA recommends three servings of whole grain cereals each day. Oatmeal certainly qualifies. It is cholesterol free and is low in total fat and saturated fat. Taken along with a healthful diet, it can help lower the nasty LDL and thus be a step in the right direction in the prevention of heart disease. It has a low glycemic index and thus will protect you from those deadly blood sugar spikes.

A bowl for breakfast is a great way to start the day when combined with fruit and juice!

Dietary Fiber

With our present lifestyle, we might well not get enough fiber to obtain the benefits that it can afford. Some of the fibers that we are discussing are not soluble in water, and others are soluble. The insoluble fiber cannot be used by bacteria, so it is not a gas producer. The soluble fiber, however, can be used by bacteria, so gas and bloating may be a problem.

The insoluble fibers go through the digestive system and create bulk for the bowels. This provides more regular bowel movements, and because it moves things along, prevents a lot of contact with irritants that might cause inflammation and cancer. (See "Bad Stuff From Grilling" chapter.) Insoluble fiber is found in wheat, rye, bran, and other grains.

Soluble fiber does dissolve in water forming a gelatinous substance in the bowel. It reportedly can bind up cholesterol and remove it in the BM. It has been found to lower the blood cholesterol by 10-15%. It is found in oatmeal, oat bran, fruit, psyllium (Metamucil, Konsyl), barley, and legumes. Citracel (hemicellulose) and FiberCon (polycarboxisal) can also be used.

Bran cereal seems to contain the greatest amount of fiber. Some brand names include: All Bran, 100% Bran, Bran Buds, Oat Bran, Raisin Bran and oatmeal. One-third cup of most of the brans contains around 8 gms of fiber. Compare this to Grape Nuts 1.4 gm, Cheerios 1.1 gm, 10 peanuts 1.4 gm, and one slice of raisin bread 0.6 gm.

Start with small portions until your system gets used to the diet change. Drink plenty of water because these are water-absorbers.

Foods that have fiber content besides the grains include fresh fruit, prunes, raisins, apricots, carrots, turnips, potatoes, and cabbage.

Bad Stuff

If I asked you what two foods have done more harm to American health than any others, what would you answer?

I know what my answer is, and I have some pretty good reasons for that answer.

My candidates for "worst foods" are the good old Hot Dog and Hamburger.

They each have lots of problems individually, but when you think of the massive number of each consumed each year in this country, it becomes really horrendous.

Let's start with the hot dog.

Hot Dog

You may already know that hot dogs contain Nitrosamines. The following is a comment from Microsoft Encarta Encyclopedia: "Curing and smoking preserves food by removing or binding water so that it is not available for the growth of organisms. These methods impart a distinctive color and flavor to the food and, in some cases, eliminates the need for refrigeration. Some studies, however, show that curing agents such as sodium nitrite may combine with other chemicals to form cancer-causing Nitrosamines. In addition, cured products tend to be very salty, and the sodium in salty foods has been linked to high blood pressure."

If you would like an interesting assignment, try finding out exactly what was in that last hot dog that you ate. I have discussed this with folks who have worked in the factories that produce them. I have been told, reluctantly, that the "leftovers" are often included. It is very difficult to find that in print.

A hot dog contains approximately 670 mgm of sodium, and a corn dog contains approximately 973 mgm of sodium.

The maximum amount of sodium for a healthy adult per day is 2,400 mgm. This is about one teaspoon of table salt. The average American consumes 4,000 to 5,000 mgm/day of salt. People on a salt-restricted diet are advised to lower that to 1,500 mgm per day. Of course you should check with your doctor if you have a health problem that makes your salt intake important. This is very important for the person who is on a low-sodium diet for any reason, but it is also important for ALL of us because of the increase in blood pressure that it brings about. The salt actually makes your body crave water. This water is held in the circulation by the salt. This increases the volume of fluid in the body, which in turn raises your blood pressure.

As the manufacturers try to limit salt content in the hot dog, there is sometimes another substance added which is monosodium glutamate (MSG). This is a salt that is supposed to trick your taste buds. It also has many side effects. The chief ones seem to be headache and gastrointestinal symptoms. So, if you have any of these types of symptoms after eating a hot dog, you should consider MSG as a possible cause of the problem. Better yet, don't eat the hot dog.

Did you know that sugars are added to hot dogs? I found that additives include sweeteners such as dextrose, corn syrup, and sugar to make the hot dog taste "really swell." Most of us do not need the extra calories that these bring with them.

No wonder the hot dog tastes so good!

Historically, hot dogs apparently came about as a way for butchers to sell the less-desirable cuts of meat. They would grind them up, add some spices and other flavors, and place them in a casing. They would then cook them so that they were ready to eat. The additives often include cereal fillers, egg white and spices (onion, garlic, salt, pepper, etc.). This "ready to eat" part certainly fits into the American lifestyle.

Figures from the American Meat Institute in 1999 estimated that Americans would buy 20 BILLION hot dogs that year.

If you are an eater of these things, I beg you to rethink that decision. It is a real trouble food.

Pertaining to the questionable contents of the hot dog, I submit this in jest. It evidently is from a popular song of 1860.

> *Oh where oh where has my little dog gone?*
>
> *Oh where oh where can he be?*
>
> *Now, sausage is good. Baloney, of course.*
>
> *Oh where oh where can he be?*
>
> *They make them of dog, they make them of horse,*
>
> *I think they made them of he.*

Sorry about that.

Hamburger

My other "worst food entry" is the hamburger. Again because each hamburger is so bad and because of the massive quantity of this meat that Americans eat. McDonald's alone at this moment is advertising that they have sold 99 BILLION hamburgers worldwide.

The hamburger has a problem of fat and cholesterol content, and for most individuals, it has a salt (sodium) problem.

As you go to the grocery store, you will find the fat content of hamburger ranges between 5% (low fat) and 30% (maximum allowed). Of course, the higher the fat content the "juicier" the hamburger. You have already realized that the leaner the product the more it costs.

There is also the problem of carcinogens. (See "Bad Stuff From Grilling" chapter.)

The Fast-food Breakfast

Breakfast could well be our most important meal of the day. It is wise to start the day right! Folks who skip breakfast usually end up with symptoms of one sort or another.

We have already mentioned the importance of "inflammation" as the cause of many of our artery problems. Researchers at Buffalo University found that the "Egg McMuffin and Hash Browns" for breakfast was really bad news for the arteries. What these researchers did was give nine normal weight individuals a glass of water after an overnight fast, and then they did successive blood sampling over the next three hours. At the same time they also took eight normal weight subjects and after an overnight fast gave them a breakfast of "Egg McMuffin and Hash Browns." They then did the successive hourly blood testing. This combination was calculated as supplying 900 calories of high-fat food for each of these eight individuals.

They found that this 900-calorie, high-fat meal temporarily floods the blood stream with inflammatory materials, which overwhelms the body's normal mechanisms for fighting the inflammation.

Levels of the inflammatory factors remained elevated for three to four hours after the high-fat meal.

The investigators felt that people who repeatedly do this to their arteries may end up with a chronic inflammation in the arteries that could be important in the development of hypertension, obesity, and atherosclerosis.

Think about this the next time that you drive by a fast-food place at BREAKFAST TIME.

Trans Fats

These are real nasties. They came about as an answer to a problem in the food industry.

They have created a terrible problem in the health of humans. When foods such as cookies are made with ordinary oils, they tend to have a short shelf life. Spoilage is a major problem for the food industry. To solve this problem, trans fats were created in the laboratory. In the process of making a trans fat, the fat is heated; at which time, bad things happen. Actually a hydrogen atom is hooked onto the fat when it is heated. The term for this process is "hydrogenation." The finished product is as harmful or more harmful to our bodies than saturated fats would be. It has become enough of a problem that the Federal Government mandated that by January 1, 2006 the amount of trans fat be labeled on each food product. As soon as the FDA set that time limit, the affected companies began trying to reduce the amount of trans fat in their foods, which is a good thing. Of course, those that have no trans fat in their products were quick to state so in their labeling.

The terms that we need to continue to look for are: "hydrogenated" and "partially hydrogenated." Unfortunately, as you look at the labels regularly, you will see these terms pop up awfully frequently. So, in your mind, you can pretty much equate trans fat, partially hydrogenated fats, hydrogenated fats, and saturated fats as being equal trouble to your body.

The stuff is everywhere. About 40% of the fat in US donuts, fries, store-purchased cookies, crackers, and margarines contain trans fats. You have to be vigilant in looking at labels and watch for little tricks. Some products will advertise that they have "reduced fats" but "lo and behold" there lies trans fat waiting to get you.

The *New England Journal of Medicine* ('99-6-24) states that there is no nutritional excuse to hydrogenate anything ...and many reasons not to.

French Fries

French Fries start with a problem and that is that a potato is a starch. This means that even before it leaves your mouth an enzyme begins converting it into sugar. It turns out then that it is sort of like eating a candy bar. There are some other problems, however. When these potatoes are boiled in oils, there is a possibility that a chemical called Acrylamide might be formed. This chemical is known to cause cancer in rats. Investigations are still going on as to whether humans can get cancer from them.

But again, this is one more instance that when you use high temperatures on fats really bad things happen. This is one more chemical to worry about. When one sees all the cancers around, one certainly has to entertain the possibility that these products may be responsible for some. There are some estimates that 30% of all cancers are diet-related.

Calorie-wise, a small bag of McDonald's Fries has 210 calories; a large bag, 540 calories; a super-size bag, 610 calories. *Source: McDonald's*

Vegetable Oil

These contain only calorie-rich fat that will be converted to body fat and cholesterol by the liver. There are many healthful substitutes on the market so that vegetable oils really are no longer needed in the kitchen.

Dark Chocolate (The Mayans called chocolate the "Food of the Gods")

After eating chocolate you feel godlike, as though you can conquer enemies, lead armies, entice lovers.

Emily Luchetti

Does one list this as a terrible food or a good food? I guess it is both. It can give you the high rises in blood sugar that we are desperately trying to prevent. It is estimated that in the US the average chocolate consumption per person per year is 11.1 pounds. We hear a lot about the benefits of chocolate, and we all know "The Devil Made Me Do It" Syndrome that happens when we pig-out and gain weight as a result.

Chocolate contains saturated fat, but about one-third of it is in the form of stearic acid that does not raise LDL and is converted in the liver to oleic acid that is a monounsaturated fat, which is heart-healthy and which the body needs.

The chocolate that we buy has sugar added, so watch your labels.

Well, anyway, the flavonoids in the chocolate are what we are interested in. There is a particular flavonoid in dark chocolate called epicatechin that is the especially beneficial part of the chemical compound.

Dr. Engeler out of the University of California did some research that turned out to be very interesting. She divided a group of subjects into two groups. She gave one group chocolate with flavonoids, and the other group got chocolate without flavonoids. After an extended period of time, it was found that the flavonoid group had less stiffness of the arteries than the other group. This is important because stiffness of the arteries is one of the early signs of artery problems leading to atherosclerosis. The flavonoids are responsible for causing some reduction in the nasty LDL, act as antioxidants, reduce the risks of blood clots, and slow down the immune response that helps lead to atherosclerosis plaque formation. Previously, about half of the flavonoids were lost in the chocolate manufacturing processes, but now about ninety-five percent of the flavonoids are retained in dark chocolate.

Dr. Engeler states that there is more flavonoid in dark chocolate than in green tea, black tea, red wine, or blueberries.

As you look over the foods listed above, you can get an idea of which foods my patients have most satisfactorily used in improving their health status. If you are ready to change your dietary ways, please take a look at the Mediterranean Diet. The people in the Mediterranean area of the world are known to have a reduced coronary artery risk compared to ours. It has now been shown that this diet can successfully be adapted in other parts of the world with similar results. The study that looked at this question was reported in the *British Medical Journal* in July 2005 (EPIC–elderly). The study took place in nine European countries and did show that the people who were following the Mediterranean Diet did live longer than those who were not following it.

The Mediterranean Diet essentially consists of a high intake of vegetables, legumes, fruits and cereals. It encourages the use of fish in the diet. It also encourages the use of olive oil, an unsaturated fat (that's good). Other foods that qualify are in the polyunsaturated and monounsaturated fat groups. These were allowed in the study in place of olive oil. Most of your food labels will advise you of the kinds of fats with which you are dealing.

So, the word right now is to avoid, if possible, the saturated fats and the trans fats, which includes hydrogenation in any form.

The Mediterranean Diet also suggests a moderate intake of alcohol. In this study, wine was used, but many other studies have now suggested that other kinds of alcohol can be substituted for wine with no lessening of the health benefit. Please remember that this benefit is for ONE or TWO drinks per day. We all know the evils that happen when people imbibe a lot. The body, family, and society suffer from that. And, remember that "one or two drinks per day" should be AFTER you have hung up your car keys for the day.

The following examples are included because of the obvious influence that both diet and exercise had on the people that were involved.

The other day I was waiting for my wife on one of her mall shopping trips. (My wife loves malls. This allows me much time to consider the problems of the world while I wait in our car for her return.) I noticed two boys in a nearby park. They were about ten years old and, unfortunately, each qualified as "fat." As I watched, I wondered what had gone wrong. They were sort of exploring some slides that were meant for much younger kids…the slides that you find…in bright colors at some deadly fast-food houses. The kind that are meant to lure the child…thus placing pressure on the parent. I wondered if these boys' parents were overweight too. I wondered how much TV per night the parents allowed. (Was there a limit?) I wondered if junk food was available during TV watching. I know one thing for certain. Both of these boys have highly increased risks of developing early heart disease, and if their parents are overweight, the chances are very slim, indeed, that they will ever be able to shed those pounds. Because of their bad habits they will be at increased risk of developing diabetes, hypertension, and a host of other problems including heart disease. I have yet to see a turnaround in kids with this magnitude of problem. In my practice I have lectured the parents of similar kids. I have also lectured the kids, sent them to dieticians, etc., but have had little success in changing their lifestyle.

What a pity!

Now, contrast that with this.

My wife and I were hiking on a mountainous trail this summer in Cumberland Falls State Park, which is located in southern Kentucky. If you haven't been there and you like to hike, you really owe it to yourself to go. The temperature was 96 degrees, and we were perspiring and drinking lots of fluids so as to be able to complete the trail on our own two feet and not be carried off on a stretcher…when to our surprise we were confronted with a beaming four-year-old little girl…on the trail…hand in hand with her mother. This child was obviously having the time of her life on this miserable (all in how you look at it, right?) day. Her mom was slim and in her late twenties. I commented to this mom on how the child was handling these adverse conditions on the trail that day. Her reply, "We like to start them out early."

And, wow, were they ever!

The very special thing about this was that the child was enjoying a beautiful day with her mom…doing stuff that mom thought was great...so, obviously, it WAS great. "To heck with the heat and steep climbs. We are having fun!" This child is well on her way, at four years of age, to having a healthy lifestyle. Her role models are superb. She will hit the salad bar first, as she obviously is already doing, and as is her mother. I am sure that that child was carried back up the trail on the return trip, but I would wager that, given a couple more years, she will make the whole trail on her own.

It has been found that children who drink more than three servings of milk per day gained more weight than those who drink fewer glasses per day. This was independent of whether it was whole milk, 2% milk, or skim milk. Some researchers think that the estrones (hormones) and whey in milk may cause weight gain. If that happens to turn out to be the case, watch out for the whey. It has crept into some of the most unlikely places. As you do your shopping, keep an eye out for it.

Let me accompany you to the food market and suggest some things to look for and why.

I encourage you to check out ingredient labels if you are not doing that already.

Let's take a look at a loaf of bread.

This loaf has outside labeling in bold letters NO TRANS FATS. (That's a good start.) The baker is well aware that you are more likely to make a purchase now, being the wise shopper that you are.

...100% whole grain. That's great. The fiber included with the "whole grain" makes it an especially healthful food. Milled white flour is nearly as harmful as sugar is in raising your blood sugar level. Whole grains get picked up by the body much more slowly and thus are slower in raising your blood sugar level. (See upcoming "Glycemic Index" section.) This avoids the sharp spike in blood sugar that is so deadly to our systems.

...No artificial colors or flavors (great...the less junk added to our food the better for us).

...Also stated is the fact that it is made with honey. Think about whether this has increased the calories per slice. The bread will certainly be sweeter for having it there, but you have to decide if the calories are for you.

Under "nutrition facts" it states that:

…Serving size is two slices. I would hope that ordinarily YOUR serving size would NOT be two slices. Cutting back on the amount of bread eaten is a good first step in reducing total calories in watching your weight.

…It states that each slice has one gram of sugar…about 4 calories. Incidentally, you may be interested in knowing that a common meal for some 600-pound persons is a LOAF of bread.

…It has no polyunsaturated or monounsaturated fats. (We need some of those, so we will have to eat our olives.)

…Sodium content is 115 mgm/slice. (It's pretty difficult to find low-sodium bread…so you have to depend on eating less in order to keep your blood pressure down where you would like it to be.) The "no-sodium" is available for a price.

Let's check out a bottle of olives.

Olives have been a major staple of the Mediterranean Diet. Let's take a look to see how it would fit into your diet. The particular brand that I am examining is very cheap. It has about 5 calories per olive so that should not be a problem. It has about 1 gram of fat per olive, but this is polyunsaturated fat, so that is good. It has no saturated fat or other fats and is free of trans fats. It doesn't supply sugars, fiber, or carbohydrates. As for sodium content, each olive contains about 60 mgm. So, unless you are on a very sodium-restricted diet, you can afford to eat several olives per day.

In summary: Olives and olive oil provide an excellent source of "polyunsaturated fat" to your diet. What is the importance of that? Researchers at Boston University found that people with arteriosclerosis have low levels of the essential fatty acids "linoleic" and "linolinic acid." They suggested that failing to meet your needs for polyunsaturated fats may raise your cholesterol level and cause heart attacks as much as eating too much fat and cholesterol products.

Psychological Aspects of Eating

We all know that our eating is influenced by things other than "hunger" or "need." The commercial advertisers are certainly aware of this. We face an onslaught daily of pictures of delectable foods prepared in tantalizing ways and with the assumption that if you eat them your rewards will be many and varied. (The couple on the Hawaiian beach sipping on a brand-name drink, for instance.)

Many people find that eating is one way to combat a stressful situation. Of course, realizing that, we must find other ways of dealing with those stresses. The odors in the kitchen fire up our appetites and may well influence us to make some unwise choices in foods in both specific food and the amount that we consume. In the upscale restaurant, the soothing music, attractive environment, and great service all can easily influence what and how much is eaten.

For some great diet suggestions and exercise advice, I would suggest that you check out Dr. Gabe Mirkin and his wife on the Web. They can be found at www.drmirkin.com.

Glycemic Index

You will come across the term "Glycemic Index." Several of the popular diets use this as their justification for being healthful diets and as an aid in losing weight. It is a ranking of carbohydrates based on their immediate effect on blood glucose levels. If the carbohydrates break down quickly and get into the bloodstream quickly, they have a higher glycemic index number. The blood sugar rises more quickly with some foods than with others. The Glycemic Index places these foods into categories such that you can tell how much or how little of a problem there is with any particular food.

This rise in blood sugar brings about a response from the pancreas to release insulin to bring the blood sugar down. If the amount of sugar is large and is taken up by your gastrointestinal tract rapidly, the insulin release is large in response. As the blood sugar falls as a result of the insulin activity, the body senses that the blood sugar now is going to go too low. The body then calls upon the liver to respond by releasing glucose to bring the sugar level back up. If the liver is not able to respond quickly, the person is in a state of "hypoglycemia" and feels "bad." Having a low blood sugar brings on sweating; your heart pounds, and you feel very weak and tired. The cure? Another bottle of pop or another candy bar, thus resulting in added pounds.

So you can see that people who eat high carbohydrate diets such as these can get into a state where their sugars are bouncing up and down all day long and they feel lousy.

The way out of this is to avoid high calorie carbohydrates. That is where the glycemic index comes in. Actually, if people are feeling THAT bad, they should follow the index numbers in choosing foods but also eat about five small meals a day until they are feeling better. Dividing up their calorie intake in this manner gives a smoothing out of blood sugars and thus a smoothing out of insulin output by the pancreas. The result in how one feels is dramatic and is overnight.

You have had a hypoglycemic episode I am sure. Everyone has had one. Think about the time that you might have skipped breakfast...worked really hard...and then felt woozy, sweaty, heart pounding, and lightheaded. Hopefully you sat down, got something to eat, and felt better. That is the way hypoglycemia works. If it doesn't go away, you should see your friendly doctor and get some testing.

The glycemic index arbitrarily assigns glucose the number 100. So that if a food releases its calories more slowly and in a lesser amount the number is set lower than 100. Alternately, if the release is faster than that of glucose, the number assigned to that food will be greater than 100.

Examples...some of which are surprising:

rye flour bread...60-80

white bread...100

whole wheat bread...90-95

Kellogg's All-Bran...40-60

oat bran cereal...60-70

Cheerios…110

Grape Nuts…95

Corn Flakes…125

brown rice…70-90

instant rice…90-120

pasta-type foods…60-70

peas and beans…35-70

banana bread…65-75

oatmeal cookies…70-80

graham crackers…105

So, what do we see at work here?

The more refined a product, like bread, the less healthful. Beans and peas are great nutritionally and also have good glycemic index numbers. Some of the very refined and messed-with cereals are not very good health foods. In fact they are lousy as health foods. But, they still beat out the Fast-Food Breakfast!

Foods with high indexes would include most breakfast cereals; processed bake goods including those great-tasting donuts, bagels, croissants, and rolls; some potatoes; table sugar; ice cream; white bread and candy.

Foods included in the lower-index group would include all of the vegetables. Whole grain foods qualify as well as most dairy foods. Fats slow down the uptake of the carbohydrate.

Fruits range from 40-80 on the scale, so some are low and some are not so low, with bananas and raisins on the high end.

No one is expected to memorize all those numbers, but if you have in your mind some generalizations about which food fits where in the index, it should help you feel better in the long run as you translate this knowledge into changes in your daily eating habits.

Along the same line, remember that if you eat a fiber food along with a carbohydrate the fiber will slow down the digestion of the carbohydrate and will act like it lowered the glycemic index of the product.

An example would be brown rice compared to white rice. White rice has the fibrous outside cover of the rice removed. The white rice will be digested much more quickly and will give a higher rise of blood sugar than if the cover were still present. All of the whole grains qualify as "good" compared to the grains that have been milled. Eating some beans along with the rice will lower the GI even more.

That Much

"That much" is the most abused phrase found in my medical practice. My patients use it daily, saying, "But Doctor, I don't eat THAT MUCH." For most people, this phrase seems to mean the amount of food that it takes to satisfy their hunger, or it may be the amount of food that they could consume five years ago and still hold their weight steady. The thyroid gland, the overseer of the body's calorie burning, has a steadily decreasing function for most of us as we age. So, unless we exercise more, we must cut back on the number of calories consumed each year or we will certainly have a weight gain. And when the 300-pound person who just gained 20 pounds in the past month says that he/she doesn't eat "that much," "that much" is certainly "too much." In my practice, "that much" is too much for most of us.

Haven't you gone to the great buffet restaurants where there is a fixed price and you can eat all you want of anything you want? I love them. When traveling, my wife and I are prepared in case we don't find one at mealtime. We have our food chest packed with ice and healthy foods. We love to picnic and have spread our lunches out on the concrete slabs of rest areas on multiple great trips. We count some of those times as some of the most memorable times of our lives. Examples: picture wind-whipped clothes...hang on to your hat...while taking in the Grand Tetons, or picture a quiet sunshiny day overlooking the Rio Grande in Texas...while eating our tuna sandwiches and chomping on our carrots.

Getting back to the buffet restaurant. I am sure that you have watched with fascination which person picks what food first. One can pretty well predict who will hit the salad bar first and who will hit the mashed potatoes and gravy with two desserts. Our natural instincts tell us to eat fatty and high carbohydrate foods. These are associated with survival instincts from at least back in the caveman days. Back then, there might not have been a meal again for another few days, so this had better be a good one. How, then, was the salad bar visitor able to override this basic instinct? I think you will agree that good role models, good education, and a desire to be really healthy have to have played a large part. What part of the buffet restaurant do YOU hit first?

So how do we know if what we eat is too much? The scales do not lie. If you are aiming for a five-pound weight loss over a two-week period, you really ought to be weighing yourself at least every other day so that you can make adjustments to your diet accordingly. As far as I am concerned, the "quickie" diets proposed by the published doctors and others are NOT the way to go. These authors are making a bundle of bucks off their products, but I have yet to see a single patient who could stick with one of these diets for even one year. And, good people, we are talking about a LIFETIME here. It is very hard on your system to get into the gain-lose-gain mode.

Good health and staying fit, including proper weight, are forever.

Rewards

Unfortunately, many people eat unwisely as a "reward" for doing so well on their diet. They feel that they "deserve" this break in the monotony of eating healthful foods. When I see this pattern, I look closely at how they are doing. If, indeed, their weight goals are being met and their lipid panels are staying where we want them to be, I do usually approve this practice. But, the majority of the time, I find that the goals are not being met, and the patient will be advised that busting their diet must cease on those occasions.

One way to do this has been to try harder to have the healthful foods NOT be boring and to be more inventive in arranging the health-food menu. I must suggest that this is a private matter for you. Your doctor can suggest a good dietician to help you through this phase if you are having a really bad time of it.

Let's examine the "reward" and see if it isn't an excuse to eat the bad stuff that the body craves so much. First, you must understand that the bad stuff really tastes good. The body craves it and objects, like everything, when it is denied. The fats and the sweets are therefore real problems that are in the way of getting where you want to go.

I do not believe that you will be able to depend on the presence of someone else to goad you into eating properly. This should be a personal matter, and you should be supplying your own reward. As you pass up the dessert or say "no" to the mashed potatoes and gravy, you must consciously or unconsciously pat yourself on the back and chalk one up for the "good guys." And, after awhile, this can get to be a habit. It should become a habit that perseveres in spite of what others around you are doing. After all, it is you, not them, that is in charge of your body. You must really take charge! We are in this thing as individuals. It is ME not THEM that will suffer the heart damage if things do not go well.

It is great when a spouse or significant other is understanding and helps in this process of reward, but again, I believe that you must plow on and stick to your dietary goals even in the face of a lack of support from the persons around you. Again, it would be you, not them, who will be in line to reap the reward or to pay the price.

Do I practice what I preach? You bet I do! If a meeting has food on the menu that doesn't qualify as fit for MY body, I have no qualms at all about eating at home before I go.

Rude? Yep.

Smart? Yep.

In fact, I did complain to the manager of a four-star hotel when a dining brunch-type table failed to include healthful foods. To find healthful food, I had to walk four blocks in the snow. Actually, the exercise was good for me. I was offered a free night's stay at the hotel, which I turned down.

Chapter 10—Exercise

Strength is the capacity to break a chocolate bar into four pieces with your bare hands—and then just eat one of the pieces.

Judith Viorst

Let's face it. Exercise is work, and it takes some motivation to start it and then to keep going with it. It is very easy to find some excuse for not doing it.

It is estimated that, in the US, less than one out of four people do enough of the right kind of exercise to affect their cardiovascular system beneficially. We really need to do better. The American Heart Association has added exercise to the list of risk factors for heart disease, along with diabetes, smoking, cholesterol, and the rest of it. It is an EQUAL part, showing how important it is felt to be. Just think, getting the right amount of exercise is as important as controlling your blood pressure. We all really do have to change our ways in light of that finding! At the present time the minimum amount of exercise per day to qualify as being enough for cardiac benefit is 30 minutes. This doesn't have to be all at one time. You could do three 10s or two 15s. However, calorie burning increases when the body heats up and when you "work up a sweat." So keep this in mind, as you plan your activities.

What a neat habit to get into!

As you begin to explore what makes a good exercise, you must make sure that whatever level of exercise you choose is appropriate for your particular level of fitness. It would be a good idea to get a checkup from your friendly physician if that hasn't happened in a while. You must advise him/her about what you are planning to do and get his/her opinion about whether that is risk-free for you.

Walking is turning out to be a very satisfactory way of exercising the body. You have seen those healthy-looking ladies doing their daily walks, swinging their arms as they go. They are swinging their arms for a reason. There are studies that show the level of cardiovascular fitness is considerably improved by just adding that movement. I see one particular walker that is continually checking her watch at various parts of her fixed course. She is checking herself against the clock. This ensures her that she is at the level of exercise that she wishes to be. My patients who are walkers have their distances measured out around town, and on bad weather days, they walk in the malls. They do not miss a day! Many of them have used this exercise to bring down weight, blood pressure, blood sugars, and cholesterol values.

Why do these folks apparently really get a bang out of doing this?

There is a reason. Our bodies have a built-in rewards system. When one gets to a particular level of performance, which usually means "really pushing it," the brain releases a chemical called an "endorphin." This endorphin gives the athlete the zing that he needs to keep practicing, forgoing other pleasures or pursuits to experience it again and again. It gives an experience similar to the "high" that one gets in certain drug-induced "highs," but is perfectly legal. It is obvious that my "regular" walkers are exercising hard enough to get the endorphin kick.

You can't beat that! The motorcycle riders and other thrill-seekers apparently get the same high in doing what they do.

Example #1: We do not have a motorcycle helmet law in Indiana, so in our larger hospitals there are a considerable number of comatose patients, many of whom have head injuries from motorcycle accidents. Guess what the nurses on those wards say is the first thing the riders ask about when they come out of their comas?

Well, what do you think they ask?

The answer:

"How is my motorcycle?" When able, they go right back to it, and for the most part, without a helmet! Talk about being hooked on the endorphins!

Example #2: Recently a skydiver's two parachutes failed to open completely. The diver hit the ground at about fifty miles an hour. The person got all busted up ending up with surgeries galore. Going back to skydiving? Can hardly wait!

What kind of exercise makes a good cardiovascular exercise?

Well, tennis isn't one of them. In tennis, you don't have a sustained movement pattern. You wait for the other guy to hit the ball, then run like the devil to hit it back and then stand around again. This pattern is repeated over and over, and if one does it long enough, one certainly can get tired and can burn a considerable number of calories. There are some things that one can do to increase the number of calories burned such as moving from foot to foot while waiting for the return. But it still isn't like cycling or walking where the muscles really do not get much of a chance to rest, which hopefully improves the level of the person's fitness.

When you get into regularly exercising, you do feel more "alive." You also have a feeling of accomplishment. You have made a change for the better in your life. You know it, and your body knows it. As a result, you are much less likely to "blow it" with a bag of goodies. You will hit the fridge and get that carrot instead.

With good heart conditioning, the left ventricle of the heart will actually enlarge so that it is a more efficient pump than before the conditioning. This enlargement isn't like the enlargement of heart failure. In heart failure of a certain kind called "cardiomyopathy," the heart muscle has gotten in trouble for one reason or another and the heart enlarges. The heart enlargement actually makes it so that there is not a whole lot of room for blood in this left ventricle. In other forms of heart failure, the whole heart enlarges trying to take care of the body's needs for circulation and is not keeping up, which leads to trouble.

The changes that happen in the heart with exercise tend to build a strong muscle and make more room for blood to be pumped out to the body with fewer beats. In my practice I see people who, at some time in their lives, have run track. As I do my physical exam, I am struck by the fact that their resting pulse is in the 50s. If you check your resting pulse, you will probably find it in the 70s-80s, which is sort of the average for the general (out of shape?) population. I sometimes surprise the patient and ask, "For what team did you run track?" I am correct 90% of the time. These people have very healthy hearts that just do not have to work as hard as other people's hearts to do the same amount of work. This benefit seems to hold up long after they have stopped running.

How great!

When you exercise "hard" enough to cause muscle soreness, the next day you have really caused some damage to individual muscle fibers. These fibers will toughen up and become stronger as they heal, and that's how we improve our strength. Because this damaged region needs some time to heal, it is wise not to do the same exercise every day. For instance, if you use a treadmill one day, you might think of cycling the next day.

For me, I find that I need the exercise equipment in my home, staring me in the face every day. My lovely wife has "put up" with having a treadmill and exercise bike in the house. Thus, weather cannot be an excuse. I may grumble a bit, but these pieces of equipment get used every day.

You will need to find what works best for you.

As mentioned previously, exercise has many benefits for the body. One of the main ways that it helps to prevent heart attacks and strokes is that it can lower insulin levels in the body. It is known that insulin is a problem. It is one of those substances that you have trouble living with but cannot live without. It is known that insulin has an artery-constricting property along with other problems. Thus we want to keep the blood levels of insulin as low as possible. Exercise is one way of doing this. This is how it works.

When we eat a meal, our glucose level rises which brings about a release of insulin by the pancreas in order to lower it. We do not particularly want that insulin running around.

The liver has the capability, as do the muscles, of converting glucose to a substance called "glycogen" which can be used for energy production by the muscles. When you exercise you deplete the glycogen that is stored in the muscles. This brings about a lowering of the blood glucose as the glucose is removed from the general circulation to replenish the glycogen that was used up by the muscles.

If you happen to be a runner or want to become a runner, I would suggest that you check out a physician's website. Dr. Gabe Mirkin and his lovely wife, Diana, run this site. Gabe is a runner and, not typical of most doctors who give diet and exercise advice, LOOKS like a runner. He and his wife will answer questions, and they do have a newsletter. These two people offer valuable information concerning healthy foods, exercise and a healthy lifestyle. They can be found at www.drmirkin.com. They also have a book published titled *The Heart Healthy Miracle* that would be an important addition to your library.

Inflammation

As research continues into the causes of the major problems that our bodies seem to experience, "Inflammation" is coming across as being a major culprit. It seems that heart disease, cancer, and even the dementia of Alzheimer's disease are associated with or caused by this process in some way. As discussed earlier, the risk of colon cancer increases with the colon's contact with toxins of the cooking and grilling of meats. It is probably going to turn out that these chemicals set up an inflammation in the cells lining the colon. This toxic contact causes the cellular changes and cellular damage that create the beginnings of a cancer. We know that anti-inflammatory drugs, aspirin for example, can reduce the risk of cancer of the colon. An antioxidant, vitamin C, also has been shown to reduce the risk of colon cancer presumably by slowing down this "oxidation" process.

Then, think of smoking. Almost all of the systems in the body are affected by smoking. Smoking is known to increase the risk of most all the cancers found in the body. Chronic obstructive pulmonary disease (COPD), which most people have begun by the time they have smoked for five years, certainly rears its ugly head as one example of chronic inflammation in action.

Inflammation in the body can also be caused by obesity, infection, allergy, surgery, hypoxia (low oxygen level), trauma, malignancy, and autoimmune disease (the inflammatory rheumatoid-type problems).

We have a few lab tests that show that the inflammation is going on, but we are not quite sure what to do with them as yet. The C-Reactive Protein (CRP) is the most important test of this sort at the present time. The problem with this test is that lots of things make it elevate. If you had a strep infection of the throat, the CRP would be elevated. If a person had rheumatoid arthritis, the CRP would also be very elevated.

But, the CRP is also elevated in coronary artery disease (CAD), and this has been studied a lot. So, to use it for heart problems, one really has to be sure that something else has not been responsible for the abnormal value before one can blame the CAD.

There are lots of doctors who believe that this test might be more valuable than the LDL in predicting heart problems. In fact, they believe that this test ought to be added to the laboratory blood panels that we use for our diagnosis and treatment of heart problems. So far insurance companies are not thrilled with that idea because, for one thing, we are not quite sure what to do about a high CRP value.

The people who encourage the use of the CRP more widely point out that the highest values of CRP have been found in people with the greatest number of cardiovascular risks.

On the other hand, another large study showed that you could better predict heart problems by using the blood pressure, total cholesterol, and smoking history.

So the jury is still out on just how valuable CRP is going to be in the future.

Many writers have suggested that the inflammation in the blood vessels is caused by a particular bacterium (Chlamydia Pneumoniae) that is found frequently in the coronary atherosclerosis plaques. Actually, some would like to blame ALL myocardial infarctions on this bacterium. As a result, they would recommend that we all get a course of antibiotics and eradicate these little bugs. This idea has not caught on.

There now has been two large trials completed that failed to show any benefit of routine use of antibiotics in prevention of future heart problems. There were 4,000 subjects in the trials. All of the subjects had experienced a recent coronary event. So, for the present, it appears that the use of antibiotics is not the answer to reducing inflammation in the coronary arteries.

Getting influenza vaccinations yearly has been shown to reduce the incidence of coronary artery disease. This apparently works because of the decreased inflammation in that group of people.

Three rules: I do not eat too much; I do not worry too much; and, if I do my best, I believe that what happens, happens for the best.

Henry Ford

This topic has been discussed a lot over the past several years. How much does a patient benefit from having a yearly physical examination? I, being a primary care provider, have done yearly physicals ever since I started in the practice of medicine. There are several benefits that I see come out of that exercise.

1.   The doctor gets to know the patient.

In these days of patients using the emergency room more and more for their primary care problems, I think it's pretty neat that there is a professional healthcare provider to whom you are not a number. You are a PERSON. We all object to being a number. (My wife carries this to the next level and refuses to memorize her social security number. This causes all sorts of problems.) The push on physicians now is to computerize our health records and place them on the Internet so that they are instantly available anyplace in the world at any time. With the skills of the Bad Guys seemingly improving every day, somehow I don't think that this is ready for Primetime. Yet physicians are really being pushed, with incentives, to proceed RIGHT NOW.

2.   Disease may be uncovered.

A skilled physician will watch to see how a person walks into the room and how he/she sits down on the chair. Clues can be picked up just from this movement. The manner of walking may be the only clue that there is Parkinson's disease present. Just listening to the voice will give clues to possible hypothyroidism, vocal cord nodules, or even tumors. The skin, hopefully with the shirt off, tells many tales such as possible previous sun-damage, other signs of hypothyroidism, or muscle wasting such as may be found with many other diseases.

I might say that while in China in a town of a couple million people I had occasion to visit a hospital because I was suffering from a worsening bronchitis. When the ER doctor came in to examine me, I thought that she would blow a gasket when I removed my shirt for her to listen to my chest. One does NOT remove one's shirt when in that particular hospital when dealing with that particular doctor! I actually got shouted at, and even though there was a language barrier, the meaning was very clear. Do not remove your shirt!   Sorry Doc, it's already off. The remainder of that visit remains another story for another time.

I believe in an inspection of the skin when an exam is being done. When I see it done otherwise, with the shirt on, I feel like the examiner might be a bit rushed and has a time constraint. The doctor will probably miss seeing more than the melanoma sitting on the patient's back that the patient has not been able to see. There are patients that do not want to disrobe, and that is fine, as long as they realize that a complete exam cannot be accomplished.

3.   Patients get to talk about some of their health concerns that they might not have thought important enough to make an appointment for.

For instance, they may bring up the fact that Aunt Mary was just diagnosed as being a diabetic and wonders what that might mean in their own lives.

4.   A chance to look carefully at the family history.

As you know, many of the health problems that beset us are more or less hooked into the genes. As more and more tests are available to investigate gene history, it spawns more and more questions about whether one wants to do the tests or not. For example, let's say we had a superduper test to predict whether one is going to get Alzheimer's disease. Would I want to get the test?

We have no cures at the moment. All we have at present are medications that may slow down the progress of the disease. I would have to think long and hard before I got the test. When they find a cure, THEN I will get the test.

5. Talk about testing.

If you are an established patient who has had testing before, making it pretty certain what testing should be done beforehand, it's nice to get the standard tests BEFORE the office visit. It seems like there is never enough time to talk about test results. That function is being taken over more and more by other personnel. What a pity! I think that is my job, and I love to do it. This gives a doctor an opportunity to pat the patient on the back for a job well done or a chance to do some teaching if things are not going well. That is not a job that should be passed off to a nurse, office assistant, or anyone else. That is the doctor's job. Time constraints are the killers here.

Chapter 12—Putting It All Together

Age does not diminish the extreme disappointment of having a scoop of ice cream fall from the cone.

Jim Fiebig

Heart Disease is still the number one killer in the United States for the population as a whole.

We have discussed the LDL bad stuff. This is the killer material. We know that if the good HDL is high enough the LDL will be reduced. The HDL can actually transport the fat out of cells. Now, how do we put this all together?

We have seen that the endothelium lining of our blood vessels is our guardian against invasion into the wall of the blood vessel by the dangerous LDL. I discussed some of the things that cause the endothelium to drop its barrier and allow the nasties to enter. These include hypertension, hyperlipidemia, and smoking. We do know that the endothelium is exquisitely sensitive to its surroundings.

Maybe you wondered, as I did, just how much insult from these high-fat meals it takes to cause appreciable damage to a blood vessel? We know that a SINGLE high-fat meal can set up inflammation in an artery. How about actual INJURY to that artery?

Will the vessel be INJURED by a high-fat meal once a day for a month?

Will the vessel be INJURED by a high-fat meal twice in one week?

How about a SINGLE high-fat meal? Will a SINGLE cheeseburger and fries cause injury to an artery?

Food for Thought...

One of the recurring themes that you undoubtedly have noticed is weight control. It is very difficult to get all these things working together if the weight isn't pretty much where it should be. And, where should it be?

If you have gotten well into adulthood and have kept your weight in the "normal" range, do not rest on your laurels. It has been shown that in both men and women one-half of these "normal" people will become overweight after thirty years. Further, one out of three women and one out of four men will actually become "obese." When you add these numbers to the number of people that were overweight in the first place, it adds up to the fact that darn near EVERYONE will be overweight or obese during their lifetime.

Why should this be?

Several things come into play for most people. For one, the activity (exercise) tends to decrease as we age. If you are exercising, it probably isn't quite as intense as it was a few years ago. Unfortunately, most people continue to eat about the same number of calories in spite of the decrease in activity. Another reason is that the thyroid tends to slow down so that the calories taken in are not burned quite as efficiently as one gets older. So what happens to the extra calories that are not burned? They are stored as fat.

We all need thirty minutes or more of exercise per day. Getting that exercise pays off in a variety of ways.

When a person is 100 pounds overweight, he or she qualifies as being "morbidly obese" and that means just what it sounds like it means. It means that the weight will eventually lead to the person's death. The person's death may come about because of a number of different factors, all of which are influenced by the weight. These include hyperlipidemia (cholesterol panel all screwed up), diabetes, and hypertension. But, of course, there are other things that happen as a result of the weight that affects the person's life. For example, the person's balance is going to be affected so that they will be more likely to fall and fracture a hip, which will definitely affect that person's survival.

I once was discussing the topic of morbid obesity with a grand lady in her 60s who qualified as being almost morbidly obese. She stated that no matter how much she eats "I never feel full."

I find this to be a very serious problem. I believe to overcome this she will need to put her whole heart and soul into changing her ways.

Some foods are just naturally more "filling" than other foods. Who can stop eating potato chips when they have eaten five? It would be a rare person indeed. Each chip is around 13 calories with about half of those calories coming from fat. I am a bit amazed to find that SUGAR is sometimes an additive to potato chips! Check your packaging! It is no wonder that we can't stop eating them.

You can name a number of foods that are just as difficult to stop eating. The cakes, the pies, the donuts, and the chocolates certainly qualify.

The more "filling" foods include the vegetables, fruits, nuts and cereals.

Try it yourself. See if you are not less hungry for the bad stuff if you begin your meal with the good stuff. It works.

Bad habits die hard, but they do die.

How about the lady who is 50 pounds overweight? This lady knows that she is overweight, but feels pretty good. She knows that she gets short of breath when she walks up a flight of stairs. She is hoping to drop a few pounds "when summer comes around."

This lady is definitely at increased risk from the things mentioned above, just not as much so. She must take the problem very seriously and start to correct it before the "I'll do it tomorrow" syndrome kicks in.

How about the 35-year-old man who walks in and is 15 pounds overweight? Is there a problem? You bet there is. This man, with aging, is very likely to increase that weight gain. This is the point in his life at which it is really important to change his ways and to get on track for a more healthful life in the years ahead. Then he would know that he is in a great position to face those coming years with the confidence that he has worked hard at being healthy and has attained that goal. It is very gratifying to have done things right and to have brought about changes in one's health and to be more fit as a result.

One reminder of how harmful "snacking" is between meals. When one eats a meal, the energy packets from the meal only circulate in the blood for a short time, then the body must pick up calories from somewhere else. From where does it get energy? It uses the fat stores. Snack in between meals, and the fat is allowed to remain unused. So, if you get a little hungry between meals you should mentally picture the fat stores being depleted and keep your hands off the refrigerator door!

Sometimes I have a patient in a very overweight category that I KNOW is not taking this whole thing seriously. I may have seen them REALLY misbehaving in a local restaurant. (This is a small town, you know.) I will get a little tough and say just what I think: "Now Tom, you have a little granddaughter. How badly do you want to see that little girl graduate from high school?" Or, "Gee Tom, it's pretty neat to get up in the morning and see the beautiful sunrise. How badly do you want to do this? Badly enough that you will start following my directions, stop smoking, lose weight, etc.?" (Watch out, I may be watching what YOU eat!)

I am very much aware that all of this gets monotonous, but my job is to prevent strokes, heart attacks, and death along with all sorts of other miseries, and these are the lifestyle changes that I believe it takes in order to attain that goal.

This obesity thing is getting so serious that there is now a prediction that the life expectancy in the United States will start DECLINING during the 21st century. It is blamed on the rising incidence of obesity. Obesity has increased 50% every ten years starting in 1980. The life expectancy in the US could DECLINE by five years over the next 10 years.

Schools

We are getting all sorts of warnings from all different directions concerning our children and the increasing obesity statistics. We must make a difference here. The schools often provide meals that do not follow health-food guidelines. When the schools are questioned, the reason given is that the children will not eat more healthful food. They enjoy their high-fat, high-carbohydrate meals. This HAS to be combated in the home long before the children are of school age. The children must learn very early in life exactly what makes up a healthful meal. There have been a few parents in my practice who have really practiced this. That means that candy will not be used as a reward. There will be no hot dogs, hamburgers or fries. There is no "clean plate club." In fact, the children will be praised when they stop eating when they are no longer hungry. Interestingly, these same parents are often the ones who have decided to "home school" their kids.

Is it possible to be successful in the public school situation? I think that it is. I have often advised that children carry their lunches from home rather than to eat what is being served at school. I realize that there may be a social stigma there. I also realize that my suggestion is seldom followed.

You that are parents must use your parent-teacher organizations and communicate with your school board to make these changes happen.

We have discussed the evils of obesity, but it is also important to take note that in both men and women that it is much worse to have your body fat around the abdomen than it is when the fat is more equally distributed around the body. This makes it especially important to get rid of that "spare tire" with any or all of the means that we have previously discussed.

Bad things happen, sometimes unexpectedly. We have all seen it happen. People with "normal" testing, such as I had, do have strokes, just as I did. We all know people who had their heart attack the day after getting checked out by their doctor. This includes a "normal" EKG (electrocardiogram).

I mentioned earlier that the standards of what is "normal" are being changed all the time. I think that the experts still have a ways to go. At the present time this "change" has to be done by "Trials" and their outcomes. This process takes time. So my advice to you is to hit these various numbers very hard on your own. Do not be satisfied with an LDL of 130 no matter how few your other risk factors. On the LDL, the lower the better until it is proven otherwise. At the present time there has been no problem with having an LDL of 70 as long as everything else is going okay.

The reason the "trials" didn't work for me and may not work for you is that they deal in "averages." They say that when you take ten thousand people and watch and see what happens over a number of years, that a "low risk" person may be okay with an LDL of 130. They did NOT say that there isn't one single individual in their category of "Low Risk" who has an LDL of 130 that won't have a heart attack tomorrow. So, I am saying, don't play the "averages." Shoot for the best possible numbers that you can attain in your testing. Know what the best numbers should be and don't become a statistic.

How low can the LDL go and not have a problem result?

A trial called the PROVE IT-TIMI22 treated patients very intensively in order to answer that question. In this trial 10% of the trial participants achieved LDL levels of 40 or lower! These people did not have any increased side effects from the higher doses of medications used. There were fewer heart attacks in the lower-LDL groups, but there was no difference in overall mortality.

More studies are attempting to answer that question.

Women's heart problems are underrated. One out of every three women will die of heart disease. The incidence of death for women is four times higher from heart disease than from breast cancer. We doctors have thought for a whole bunch of years that estrogen's effect on women would make these women less likely to develop heart disease.

Wrong! Their heart disease seems delayed as compared to men, but it is only DELAYED. There has been both under-diagnosis and under-treatment of women. This apparently is due to a couple factors. One, women don't seem to have the typical symptoms of heart problems as often as men do. Instead of the chest pain that comes with exercise that goes away with rest, they may have increasing shortness of breath, easy fatigability, and tiredness. They may not recognize that these are serious symptoms that need reporting. Even after the diagnosis is made, the treatments are often less rigorous and thus not as beneficial as those that the men receive. The attending doctors have to be very vigilant indeed to search out symptoms in women that may need further investigation. Unfortunately, I have seen cases where even really great cardiologists have just "missed it" on diagnosing heart disease in women. So it is important for you to be especially vigilant, if you are a female or if you have someone close to you who is a female, to keep coronary artery disease in the back of your mind to avoid tragedy.

You must, first of all, see your doctor and obtain the testing that I have discussed. You MUST know your fasting blood sugar, your serum cholesterol, triglycerides, HDL and LDL! The C-Reactive Protein would be nice, as would the homocysteine level. It has been shown in multiple studies that some patients just haven't attained their most desirable results on this testing for one reason or another. You, the patient, must educate yourself as to what your best numbers should be. You must push to be your very best. (Yes, I just repeated myself.)

Elevated levels of insulin are very harmful to our bodies, as is elevated blood sugars. The elevated sugars and insulin problems should be viewed as symptoms of a larger problem. They are definitely connected with increased levels of cardiovascular risk. The risk is increasing long before a person becomes diabetic. I am certain that blood sugars in the range that we are calling "prediabetic" will be treated with medication within a year or so. It is absolutely essential that you know that your blood sugar is in the "normal" range and, if it isn't, that you do something about it!

The HbA1c has been discussed and remains the standard measure of good diabetes control. Strive for the six range. Seven is not terrible, but eight is unacceptable. Yet there are many diabetics running around on a single medication with an HbA1c of eight or higher. This is poor control, and the body will pay the price. So, if you are a diabetic, or if your loved one is a diabetic, please push for excellent control.

The rewards are many.

Newer tests such as the CT Scans to calculate the amount of calcium in the heart vessels show great promise. At present they are not covered by insurance.

One must make a final mention of smoking as one of the greatest insults one can inflict on the human body. I was shocked to learn that the coronary arteries of aborted fetuses show signs of fatty streaking (early atherosclerosis) when the mother has been a smoker.

Certainly, if you know any pregnant female who smokes, please share this information with her.

Then, of course, smoking makes all of the other problems worse. So try to help your loved ones stop smoking if they still are. And, of course, don't stand close to a smoker and do plead your case for a smoke-free environment when you are able.

I close with these observations. I know that all of the fast-food chains have added some healthful foods to their menus. And, that's great! The fact remains that these fast-food chains still report that their bestsellers by far have been, and continue to be, burgers, fries and pizza. A blazing ad a few days ago said to the world that one fast-food chain had sold over 99 BILLION burgers!

When my wife and I visited China a few years back, we found almost a complete absence of obesity in adults and in children. The Chinese people do their exercises daily, often outside, and often in groups of forty or fifty people. They exercise religiously. They consume a lot of rice and vegetables, etc., and not much meat.

There was one place of business on our itinerary in Beijing, however, that was an exception. There, almost all of the Chinese children present were overweight. The young Chinese people seen serving the food were also overweight.

The place…

McDonald's.

I am not sure that the Big Mac was to blame…but it does make you wonder.

McDonald's Statistics:

They are sold in 122 countries around the world.

They serve from 31,000 locations.

They serve 51 million customers daily.

Source: McDonald's

References

Adams NR, McCredie R, Jessup W, et al. Oral L-Arginine improves endothelium-dependent dilatation and reduces monocyte adhesion to endothelial cells in young men with coronary artery disease. Atherosclerosis; 1997: 129:261-269.

Adler AI, Stratton IM, et al. Association of systolic blood pressure with macrovascular and microvascular complications of type 2 diabetes. BMJ 2000; 32 (7258): 412-419.

Ahmad Aljada, et al. Increase in intranuclear nuclear factor kB and decrease in inhibitory factor kB in mononuclear cells after a mixed meal: evidence for proinflammatory effect; Amer J of Nutrition. vol 79 No 4; April 2004 :682-690.

American Gastroenterological Ass. (2002) AGA technical review on obesity. Gastroenterology; 123(3): 882-932.

Anderson DC Jr. Pharmacologic prevention or delay of type 2 diabetes mellitus. Ann Pharmacoth ; 39: 102, 2005.

Antioxidants in chocolate. Lancet. Sept 1996; 348(1): 834.

Aquilera CM, Ramirez-Tortosa, et al. Protective Effect of monounsaturated fats and polyunsaturated fatty acids on the development of cardiovascular disease. Nutr Hosp. May 2001 June 30: 16 (3): 78-91.

Austin MA, Breslow TL, et al. Low density lipoprotein subclass patterns and risk of myocardial infarction. JAMA 1998; Oct 7, 260(13) :1917-21.

Barry J, Mead K, et al. Effect of smoking on the activity of ischemic heart disease. JAMA 1989;261:399-402.

Berkey C, et al. Milk dairy fat, dietary calcium and weight gain. A 543-50 longitudinal study of adolescents. Arch ped adol med; 2005: 159

Brolin RE (2002). Bariatric Surgery and long-term control of morbid obesity. JAMA; 288(22): 2793-2796.

Brown BG, Zhao XQ, Chait A, et al. Simvastatin and niacin, antioxidant vitamins, or the combination for the prevention of coronary artery disease. N Engl J Med 2001; 345: 1583.

Burr ML, Fehily AM, Gilbert JF, et al. Effects of fat, fish, and fiber intakes on deaths myocardial re: diet and reinfarction trial (DART). Lancet; 1989 :2757-761 (abstract).

Burr ML, Sweetham PM, Fehily AM. Diet and reinfarction. EU heart j.1994; 15: 1152-1153 (abstract).

Callister TQ, Raggi P, Cooli B, et al. Effect of HMG-CoA Reductase Inhibitors on coronary artery disease as assessed by electron-beam computed tomography. N Engl J Med. 1998; 339: 1972.

Cannon CP, Braunwald E, McCabe CH, et al. Antibiotic treatment of Chlamydia Pneumoniae after acute coronary syndrome. N Engl J Med. 2005; 352:1646-1654.

Danesh J, Wheeler JG, Hirschfield GM, et al. C-reactive protein and other circulating markers of inflammation in the prediction of coronary heart disease. NEJM 2004; 350:1387.

Davignon J, Ganz P. Role of endothelial dysfunction in atherosclerosis. Circulation 2004; 109:1127.

Effect of simvastatin on coronary atheroma: the Multicentre Atheroma Study (MAAS). Lancet 1994; 344:633.

Franco O, et al. Blood pressure in adulthood and life expectancy with cardiovascular disease in men and women. Life course analysis. Hypertension.

Gardner CD, Fortman SN, Krause RM. JAMA 1996 Sept 18; 276 (11): 875-81.

Grayson JT, Kronmal RA, Jackson LA, et al. Azithromycin for secondary prevention of coronary events. N Engl J Med 2005; 352: 1637-1645.

Inhibition of LDL oxidation by cocoa. Lancet, Nov. 1996; 348 (2):1514.

Koenig W, Sund MF, Rohlich M, et al. C-Reactive protein, a sensitive marker of inflammation, predicts future risk of coronary heart disease in initially healthy middle-aged men. Results from the MONICA (Monitoring trends and determinants in cardiovascular disease) Ausburg Cohort Study, 1984 to 1992. Circulation.

Konnzem SI, et al. Controlling hypertension in patients with diabetes. Am Fam Physician; 66:1209,2002.

Lewis EJ, Hensecker LG, et al. The effect of angiotensin converting enzyme on diabetic nephropathy. NEJM 1993; 329(20): 1456-1462.

Liszka, et al. Prehypertension and cardiovascular morbidity. Annals of family medicine 2005;3(July-August):294-299.

Maulaz, Alexandre Balzano, et al. Effect of Discontinuation of Aspirin on the risk of brain ischemic stroke. Arch Neurol; August 2005 62:1217-1220.

McSweeney JC, Cody M, O'Sullivan, et al. Women's early warning symptoms of acute myocardial infarction. Circulation; 2003:108.

Mirkin G, Mirkin D. The Healthy Heart Miracle.

Multicentre anti-atheroma study (MAAS); Effect of simvastinon on coronary atheroma. lancet. 1994;344:633.

Notes on smoking. The Zena and Michael A. Wiener Cardiovascular Institute and The Henry K. Kravis Center for Cardiovascular Health. Mt. Sinai Hospital; 2005.

Obrien PE, Dixon JB. Weight loss and early and late complications. The international experience. Am J Surg 2002; 184(6B): 42-55.

Ohkubo Y, Kishikawa H, et al. Intensive insulin therapy prevents the progression of diabetic microvascular complications in Japanese patients with non-insulin dependent diabetes mellitus: a randomized prospective 6-year study. Diabetes Res Clin Prac. 1995:28: 103-117.

Olshansky SJ, et al. A potential decline in life expectancy in the United States in the 21st century. NEJM. 352; 11:1138-1145.

Ramachandran S, Vasin, MD, Pencino Michael J. PHd, et al. Estimated risks of developing obesity in the framingham heart study. Ann of In Med. 4 Oct 2005; vol 143, 7:473-480.

Ridker PM, et al. Non HDL cholesterol apolipoprotein aA1 and B100, standard lipid measures, lipid ratios, and CRP as risk factors for cardiovascular disease in women. NEJM. March 2000;342:836-843.

Ridker PM, Cushman M, Stampfer MI, et al. Inflammation, aspirin, and the risk of cardiovascular disease in apparently healthy men. NEJM 1997; 336:973.

Rohde LE, Hennekens CH, Ridker PM. Survey of C-reactive protein and cardiovascular risk factors in apparently healthy men. Am J Card 1999;84:1018.

Rosenberg L, Kaufman DW, Helmrich SP, Shapiro S. The risk of myocardial infarction after quitting smoking in men under 55 years of age. N Engl J of Medicine 1985;313:1511.

Spector Tim. Obesity may accelerate the aging process; Lancet (DOI:10.1016/SO140-6736(05)66630-5).

Strong JP, Malcolm GT, et al. Prevalence and extent of atherosclerosis in adolescents and young adults. Implications for prevention from the pathobiological determinants of atherosclerosis in youth study. JAMA 1999; 281:727.

Tanne E, et al. Body fat distribution and long-term risk of stroke mortality. Stroke 2005 (May;36);1021-1025.

Trichopoulou A, et al. Modified Mediterranean diet and survival: EPIC-elderly prospective cohort study; BMJ; July 2005:271-5.

UK Prospective diabetes study group. Tight blood pressure control and risk of macrovascular and microvascular complications of type 2 diabetes. BMJ; 1998; 317: 703-713.

Wender Richard. Diabetes Type 2 Diagnosis and treatment. Temple University Family Practice Review, 2004.

Wildman Rachel P, Farhat Ghada, et al. Weight change is associated with change in arterial stiffness among young healthy adults. Hypertension 2005;45:187.

Wilson PW. Established risk factors and coronary artery disease: The framingham study. an hypertens; 1994 ; 7 : 7S.

Wiviott Stephen, Cannon Christopher, et al. Can LDL be too low? The safety and efficacy of achieving very low LDL with intensive statin therapy. A PROVE IT-TIMI-22 substudy. J Am Coll Cardiol. 46: 1411-1416.

Yusuf S, Hawken S, Ounpuu S, et al. Effect of potentially modifiable risk factors associated with myocardial infarction in 52 countries (the Interheart Study); case-control study. Lancet 2004;364:937.

Zhao HL. An update on the management of nephropathy in type 2 diabetes. J clin med ass; 66:627, 2003.

Made in the USA
Monee, IL
07 July 2026

56552251R00070